Cardiac Surgery

Acquired Heart Disease

A Colour Atlas of

Cardiac Surgery

Acquired Heart Disease

James L. Monro
F.R.C.S., Consultant Cardiac Surgeon,
Wessex Cardiac and Thoracic Centre,
Southampton General Hospital

Gerald Shore
Clinical Perfusionist, Wessex Cardiac and Thoracic Centre,
Southampton General Hospital

Wolfe Medical Publications Ltd

Copyright © James L. Monro, Gerald Shore, 1982
Published by Wolfe Medical Publications Ltd, 1982
Printed by Royal Smeets Offset b.v., Weert, Netherlands
ISBN 0 7234 0771 1 Cased edition
ISBN 0 7234 1616 8 Paperback edition
Paperback edition © 1989

For a full list of Wolfe Medical Atlases, plus
forthcoming titles and details of our surgical,
dental and veterinary Atlases, please write to
Wolfe Publishing Ltd, 2-16 Torrington Place,
London WC1E 7LT.

General Editor, Wolfe Surgical Atlases:
William F. Walker, DSc, Ch.M, FRCS(Eng), FRCS(Edin), FRS(Edin)

Contents

To our wives
Jane and Delia

Preface

Textbooks of operative surgery rarely give a true impression of what the surgery actually looks like. A collection of line drawings, often by many different artists, neither shows the surgeon how the operation is performed, nor prepares the student for what he will see. The operative photographs in this book aim to show the steps in the commoner operations performed for acquired heart disease.

There are as many different ways of doing an operation as there are surgeons; however, most operations have basic set principles. Some of the rarer operations have been excluded as this book is basically aimed at junior doctors starting cardiac surgery. From reading the relevant chapter, they should be able to understand the various steps in each operation and hopefully be a more useful assistant for having done so. It is hoped, however, that more senior surgeons will find at least some of the chapters helpful. Newly qualified doctors and medical students will be able to refer to the appropriate chapter before watching an operation and thereby better understand what they see. Nurses should benefit to the same extent and particularly operating department nurses taking cases will find the various stages of the operation set out so that they can understand what the surgeon is doing.

The text has been kept to a minimum so as not to detract from the atlas format that has been so effective in other books in the Wolfe series. Details of pre-operative assessment and post-operative care have been virtually excluded but enough references have been included to enable the reader to look further into the subject.

It must be remembered that at all times the good of the patient has come first and therefore if it would have delayed the operation unjustifiably, photography has been abandoned. The photographs in this book were taken by Mr G. Shore on Kodak Ektachrome 64 ASA 19 DIN film. The camera was an Alpa Surgical Model 81 fitted with a 50 mm f/1.9 Kern Macro-Switar lens and with an exposure setting of 1/60th second at f/22. A surgical Xenon strobe light source was used. Mr Shore is one of the perfusionists at the Wessex Cardiac and Thoracic Centre, Southampton, and has therefore been readily available to take photographs of any suitable patient. It has taken several years to collect these photographs and, in an attempt to include only clear photographs, many series of photographs have been discarded but, even so, because of limited access for certain operations, some pictures are still not as clear as they might be. However, as all photographs were taken during the course of an operation, they provide a true picture of what the operation actually looks like, even if this sometimes appears rather messy and haemorrhagic. It is hoped that the reader will soon recognise landmarks such as the sternal retractor, which is common to so many operations, and furthermore by knowing its size, be able to establish the scale. The orientation is the same throughout with the head of the patient at the top of the page.

References have been kept to a minimum and have all been grouped together in chapters at the end of the text after the last chapter.

Acknowledgements

All the photographs in this book were taken during operations performed at the Southampton Western Hospital. We are indebted to all the medical staff, operating room nurses and technicians who have been involved. In particular, we would like to thank Mr Brian Lewis (Chief Perfusionist) and Mr Charles Gilmore (Perfusionist) for standing in for Mr Shore when he unexpectedly had to take photographs. Also we would like to thank Dr John Manners and Dr John Edwards (Consultant Anaesthetists) who have graciously made room for the photographer during those operations recorded. We would like to thank Sir Keith Ross for his permission to use the photographs 15 – 21 in Chapter 5.

We would like to thank Dr Alan Johnson and Dr Neville Conway for referring the patients, also the staff of the Teaching Media Department, Southampton University for their help with developing the film.

We would like to thank Cathy Slatter, who drew the diagrams, and our publishers for their invaluable assistance and advice in the preparation of this book.

A large amount of secretarial work has been involved and we would particularly like to thank Miss Julie Poore for her cheerful and painstaking help with typing the manuscript.

1: Introduction

Cardiac surgery is still a relatively new discipline and there have been marked changes, not only in the pattern of disease treated, but also in the operative techniques and equipment available. Closed mitral valvotomy is now rarely performed in the Western world, although it is still used, for very good reasons, on a large scale in countries such as India. The many types of valve used for valve replacement bear witness to the fact that none is yet perfect. The prosthetic valves all have an incidence of thromboembolism despite long-term anticoagulation, although valve failure is now rare. The tissue valves, which have the advantage of not needing anticoagulants, still have a long-term problem of valve failure. In this book, the valves commonly used by the author are shown, although there are obviously many other alternatives available.

Whereas in the 1960s valve surgery was much the most common form of surgery undertaken for acquired heart disease, in the 1970s surgery for coronary artery disease increased enormously both in isolation and combined with other surgery. The very satisfactory results of what is, in effect, rather sophisticated plumbing, will ensure that this type of surgery will continue to occupy a very large amount of the cardiac surgeon's time.

Each chapter sets out to illustrate the different types of operation in isolation. However, frequently a combination of procedures is needed, such as multiple valve replacements, aortic and mitral being the commonest, or valve replacement and coronary artery bypass grafting. Any patient with a defect resulting from coronary artery disease, such as left ventricular aneurysm, acquired ventricular septal defect or mitral incompetence due to papillary muscle dysfunction, will frequently need a vein graft to other affected coronary arteries.

The pre-operative assessment of the patient is very important and the surgeon relies heavily on the cardiologist to provide the exact diagnosis. Furthermore, the clinical state should be as good as possible pre-operatively with heart failure adequately treated.

The patient is suitably anaesthetised and paralysed[1] and an endotracheal tube is inserted. The patient is then ventilated except when the patient is on full cardiopulmonary bypass.

The surgeon opens the chest and the vast majority of operations are performed through a median sternotomy as illustrated in Chapter 2.

Before inserting the cannulae, the patient is heparinised to prevent clotting in the bypass circuit. Once the cannulae are in position, and connected to the tubing coming from the bypass machine, cardiopulmonary bypass can be commenced. The desaturated venous blood siphons back from the patient to a disposable bubble oxygenator. Oxygen and carbon dioxide are bubbled through the blood in the oxygenator and the fully saturated blood is defoamed and pumped back by the machine to the patient. There are many different types of cardiopulmonary bypass arrangements and the reader is referred to other descriptions[2] as this is outside the scope of this book.

Once bypass has been commenced, the operation can really begin. For operations such as coronary artery surgery (see Chapter 9), the heart is not actually opened, but must be still to allow the intricate distal anastomoses to the coronary arteries to be performed accurately. Therefore, it is necessary to clamp the ascending aorta to stop the heart beating. Some surgeons then quickly perform the anastomosis and release the clamp between performing each distal anastomosis. Although the period of ischaemia does not appear to have any significant immediate deleterious effect on the myocardium if kept to less than 15 minutes, probably most surgeons, and certainly the author, prefer to protect the myocardium with the institution of cold cardioplegia.[3]

1

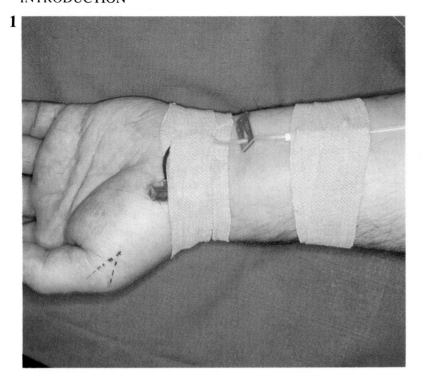

2

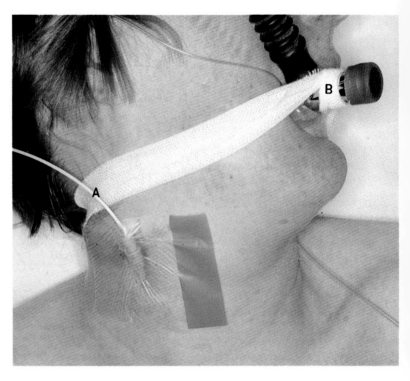

1 In order to monitor the arterial pressure during the operation, a cannula is inserted percutaneously into the radial artery, securely fixed and connected to a transducer and monitor giving a direct read out of the arterial pressure.

2 To monitor the venous pressure and for the administration of drugs, a central venous pressure line can most conveniently be inserted into the internal jugular vein (**A**). The endotracheal tube (**B**) is also seen in this picture.

3

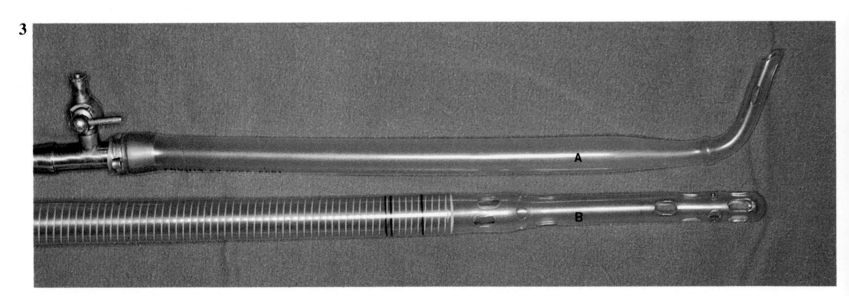

3 The types of cannulae most commonly used by the author are shown here. The arterial cannula (**A**) has a curve at the end to enable the surgeon to fix it out of the way at the upper end of the wound, and side holes to allow easier escape of blood, particularly if the end of the cannula is lodged in the left carotid or left subclavian arteries. However, many surgeons use a straight cannula and there are many different types available. The venous cannula (**B**) is, again, just one of the many types used.

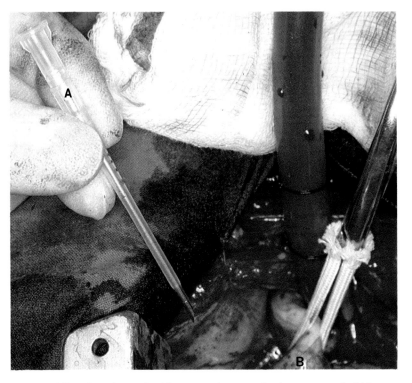

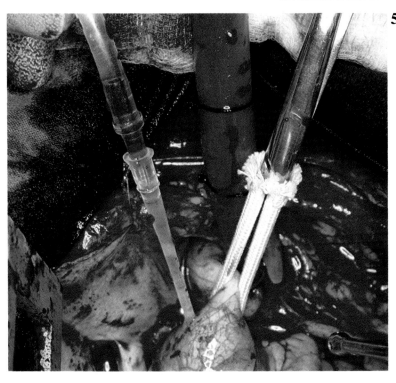

4 Providing there is no significant aortic regurgitation, a cannula (**A**) can be stabbed into the ascending aorta proximal to the aortic cross-clamp (**B**).

5 The cannula is then connected to drip tubing which has previously been filled with cardioplegic solution at 4°C and debubbled.

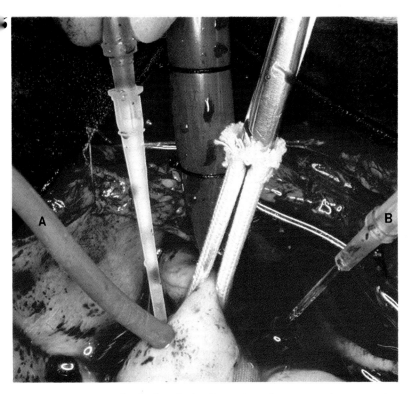

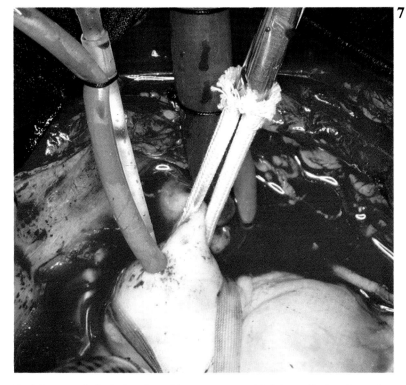

6 A litre of the cardioplegic solution is run in and a purse-string suture is placed around it and snugged on a rubber snugger (**A**). At the same time, topical cooling with cold Hartmann's solution is run into the pericardium through a separate drip tube (**B**).

7 The cannula is tied to the rubber snugger and left in until after the main part of the operation is finished, as it is sometimes necessary to give a further amount of cardioplegic solution.

INTRODUCTION

Sometimes, when there is aortic regurgitation, it is necessary to open the ascending aorta and infuse cardioplegic solution directly down the coronary arteries. This is particularly the case when aortic valve replacement is performed (see Chapter 4). An alternative method of myocardial preservation, which is applicable in the case of aortic valve replacement, is continuous coronary artery perfusion. This allows the heart to beat while the valve is replaced. However, this method has rather been superseded by cardioplegia.

For many of these operations, it is common practice to insert a vent into the heart, which is connected to one of the open-heart suckers, returning blood to the oxygenator. It is possible to insert the vent through the apex of the left ventricle (see Chapter 4) or left atrium (see Chapter 5). However, for isolated coronary artery surgery, a vent is rarely necessary and this reduces the risk of air embolism.

Air must be carefully removed at the end of any operation in which the heart has been opened. If left in the heart, it will be ejected into the aorta and may well cause a cerebral air embolus. Air may be trapped in corners of the heart, such as the left atrial appendage, roof of the left atrium or in between the muscular trabeculae in the left ventricle. It can be removed by inverting the left atrial appendage, by aspirating the roof of the left atrium with a needle, and by waiting for an adequate time during and after coming off bypass with a sucking vent attached to a needle in the aorta, while the ventricle beats more strongly.

After the main part of the operation is finished, bypass is carefully discontinued, taking care to raise the venous pressure sufficiently so that an adequate arterial pressure is achieved. If the blood pressure is inadequate at this stage, it may be necessary to give some inotropic drugs, such as adrenaline or dopamine.

After removal of the venous cannula, more blood can be given back through the arterial cannula until an adequate venous pressure is achieved. The remaining blood in the oxygenator can then be gradually run into the patient as needed, and in this way blood is saved and, indeed with care, it may not even be necessary to give homologous blood.

Once the cannulae are removed, protamine sulphate is given to reverse the heparin and the chest is closed. During this time, however, the anaesthetist must keep a constant check on the patient's progress as the cardiac output can fall, particularly in those patients who were particularly ill pre-operatively. This is only the start of the all-important post-operative care,[4] which is, however, outside the scope of this book.

2: Median sternotomy and institution of cardiopulmonary bypass

The midline approach gives excellent exposure for virtually all procedures requiring cardiopulmonary bypass for acquired disease. In this chapter, the routine procedure for institution of cardiopulmonary bypass will be described. Whether one or two venous cannulae are inserted depends on what operation is to be performed. Clearly, if the right atrium is to be opened (as for a tricuspid valve procedure), a cannula must be placed in each vena cava, and an air-tight seal must be achieved, or air will be sucked down into the venous return causing an air-lock, which will impair venous return. If the right atrium does not need to be opened (as for aortic valve replacement), one venous cannula is quite adequate. However, when the mitral valve is being replaced, considerable retraction is needed which may occlude the venae cavae, and it is therefore preferable to insert two cannulae.

Otherwise, all procedures have the same basic steps as outlined in this chapter and if the operating team follows the same routine every time, what may otherwise be a rather tedious part of cardiac surgery, can be dealt with quickly and efficiently.

1

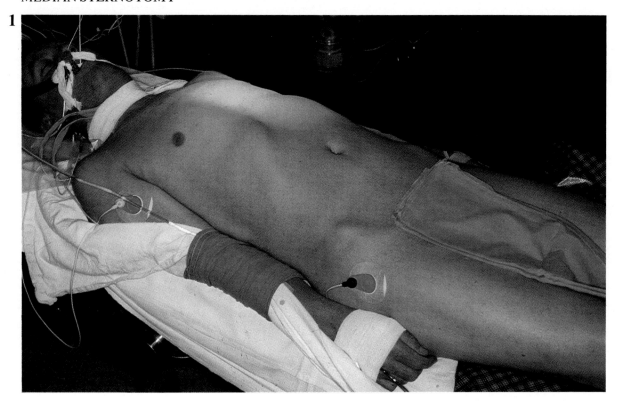

1 The anaesthetised patient is placed on his back on the operating table. The skin is prepared with iodine or some other suitable antiseptic, and this includes the legs if vein is to be removed for coronary artery bypass grafting.

2

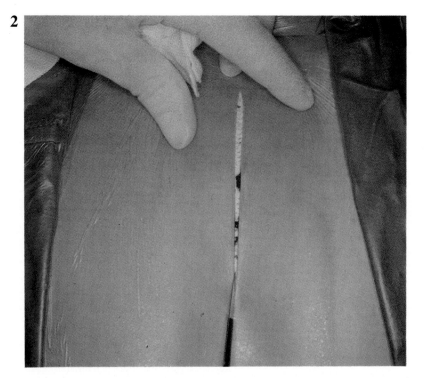

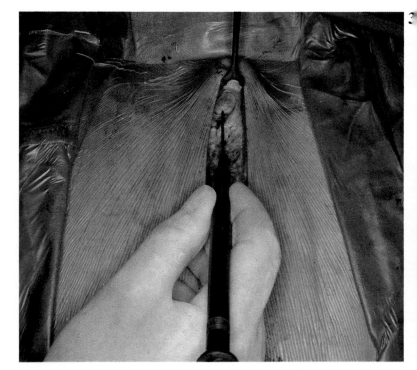

2 and 3 Drapes are placed around the chest and 'Steridrape' applied. The knife is used to incise the skin, but the deeper layers are divided down to the bone with diathermy. This minimises oozing of blood when the patient is heparinised.

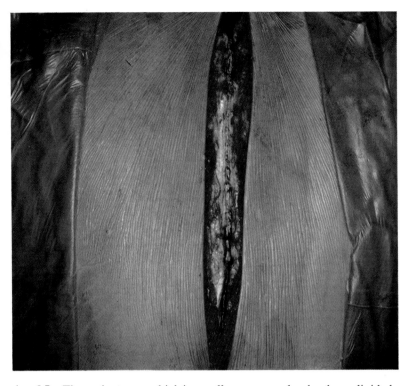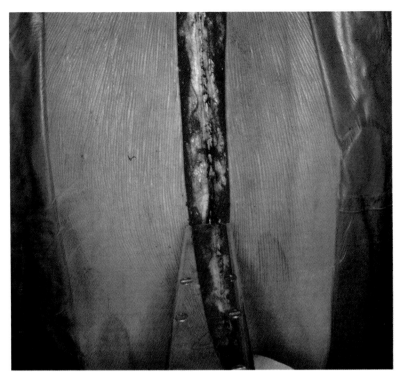

4 and 5 The periosteum, which is usually very vascular, has been divided with diathermy and the sternum is incised longitudinally with a mechanical saw.

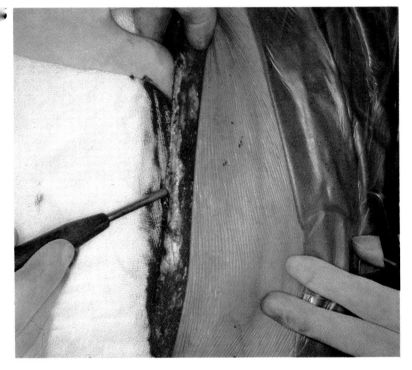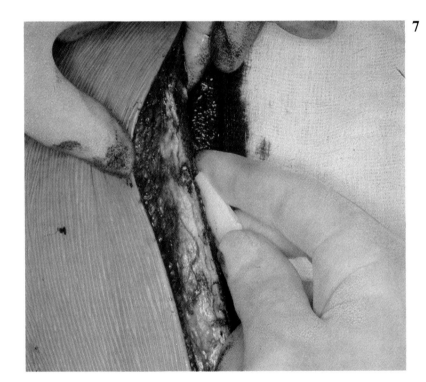

6 and 7 The sternal edges are diathermied, and wax sparingly pressed into the cut surface of the bone to stop bleeding.

8

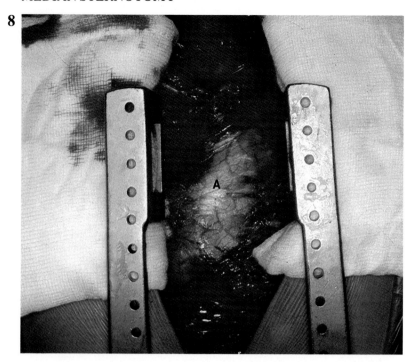

9

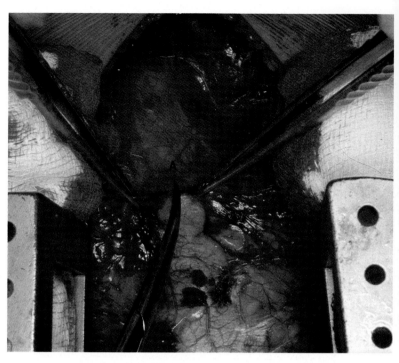

8 A swab has been placed over the bone on each side and the sternal retractor inserted. On spreading the retractor, the pericardium (**A**) is revealed.

9 It is usually necessary to divide the fat (**A**) or thymic remnant, upwards, but care must be taken not to damage the left innominate vein.

10

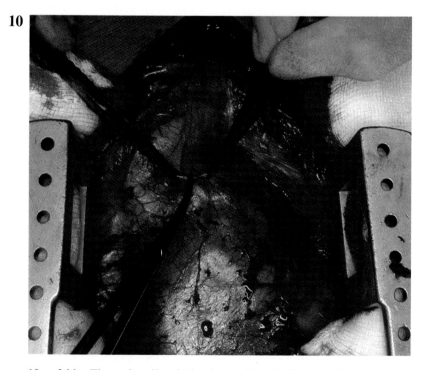

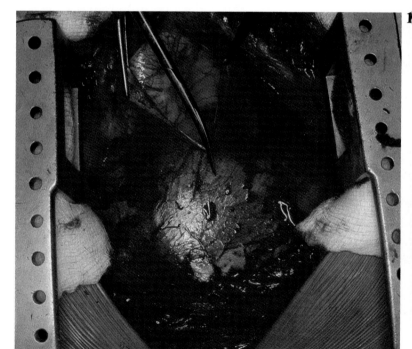

10 and 11 The pericardium is then opened longitudinally with scissors.

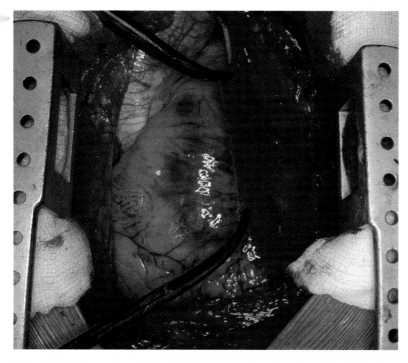

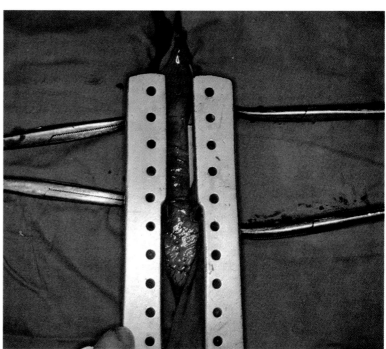

12 and 13 Two pairs of Robert's forceps are placed on the pericardial edge on either side. The swabs are replaced by side-towels, and the retractor replaced, at the same time catching the pericardial edge, held up by forceps.

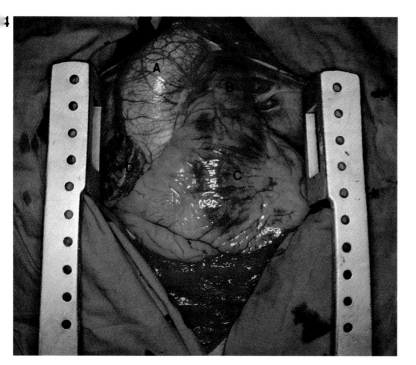

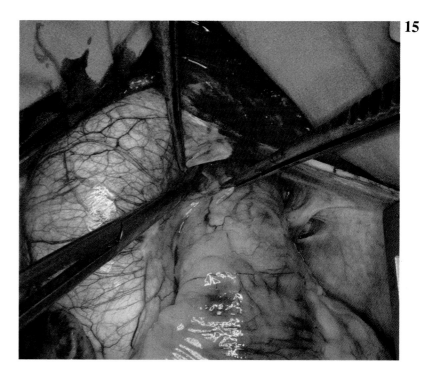

14 On spreading the retractor, the heart is revealed. The aorta (**A**), pulmonary artery (**B**), right ventricle (**C**) and right atrial appendage (**D**) can be clearly seen.

15 As in virtually all operations the aorta will be clamped, it is necessary to dissect down between the aorta and pulmonary artery.

16

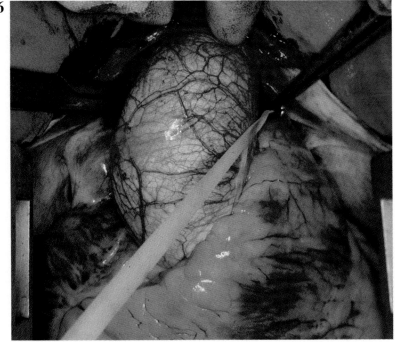

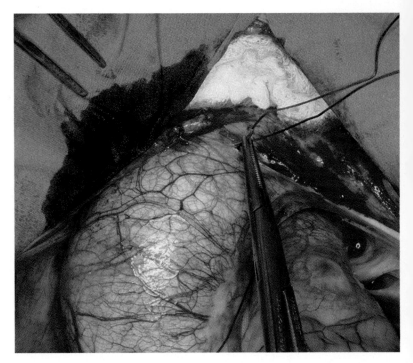

16 A tape can then be passed around the aorta at this point, which can be helpful in pulling up the aorta to make application of the clamp easier.

17 to 19 To prepare for insertion of the aortic cannula, a purse-string suture is placed in the uppermost part of the ascending aorta. It is placed just deep enough to penetrate the adventitia and part of the media, but not through into the lumen of the aorta, or a haematoma will form. If the needle is inserted only four times, a diamond-shaped purse-string is established, which is very satisfactory. The adventitia in the middle of the stitch can be cut with scissors, as this makes insertion of the cannula easier.

18

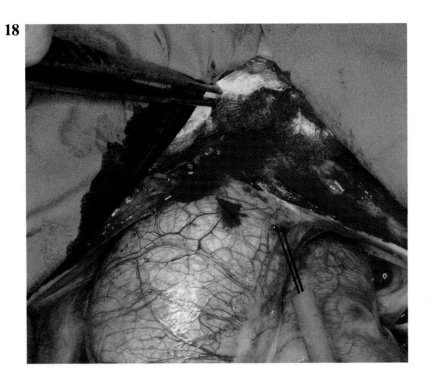

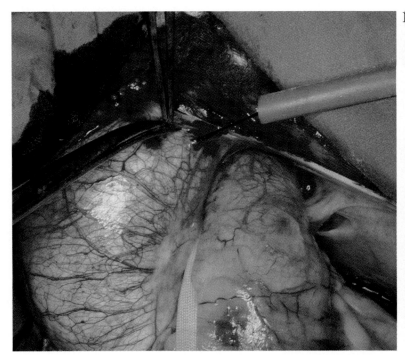

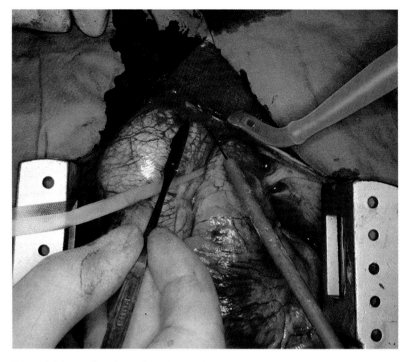

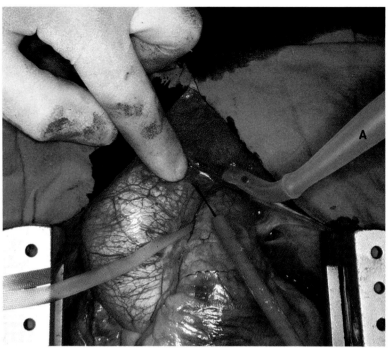

20 and 21 Before inserting the aortic cannula by this stab technique, it is important to ensure that the patient is not hypertensive. The anaesthetist should lower the blood pressure if necessary to about 100 mmHg systolic. If it is high, e.g. more than 140 mmHg, there is a considerable increased risk of causing aortic dissection. A transverse hole, just smaller than the diameter of the tip of the cannula is made with the point of the knife and a finger quickly placed over it to stop bleeding. An assistant holds the cannula (**A**) ready for insertion.

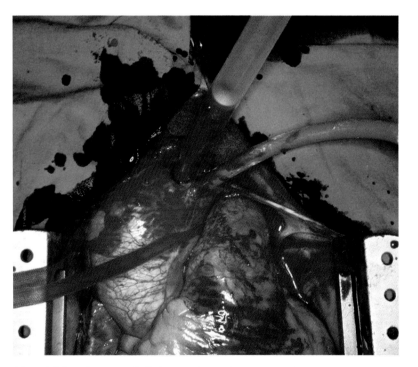

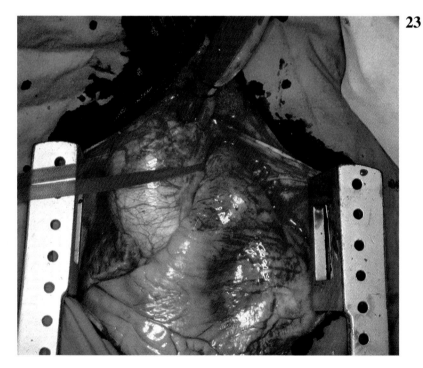

22 and 23 The cannula is inserted and the purse-string suture snugged. Blood is allowed to come up the cannula and the cannula is clamped. The cannula is then doubly tied to the rubber snugger to prevent it from being dislodged.

24

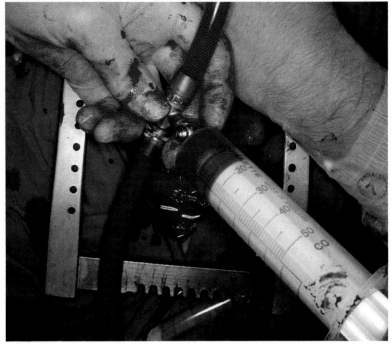

24 The aortic cannula is connected to the arterial line and air removed through a three-way tap.

25

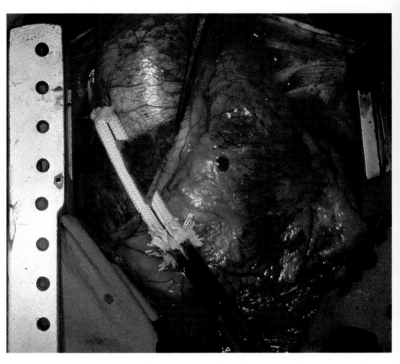

25 In preparation for insertion of the venous cannulae, a Brock clamp is applied to the right atrial appendage.

26

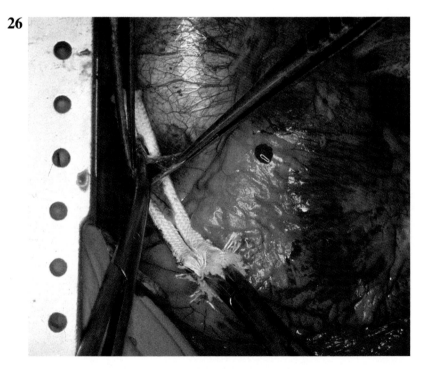

26 The tip of the appendage is cut off, and the appendage opened wide enough to allow insertion of the appropriate venous cannula.

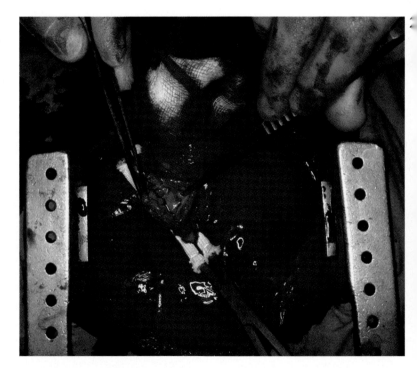

27 It may be helpful sometimes to assess whether tricuspid regurgitation is present, and this can be best achieved by inserting a finger into the right atrial appendage to feel the tricuspid valve and any regurgitant jet. In this patient, the incision of the appendage has been made large enough to accept a finger.

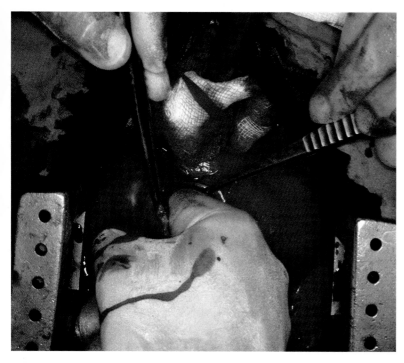

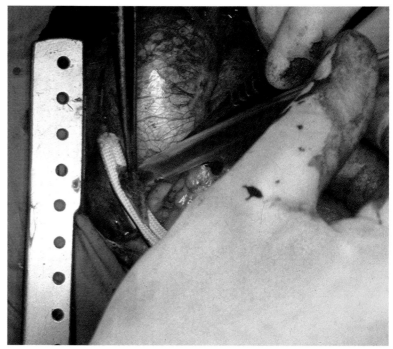

28 While the edges of the atrial appendage are held with forceps, the Brock clamp has been released and the right index finger inserted to assess the tricuspid valve.

29 to 31 The venous cannula is now placed through the right atrial appendage and passed down into the inferior vena cava. The rubber is snugged and the tube tied to it.

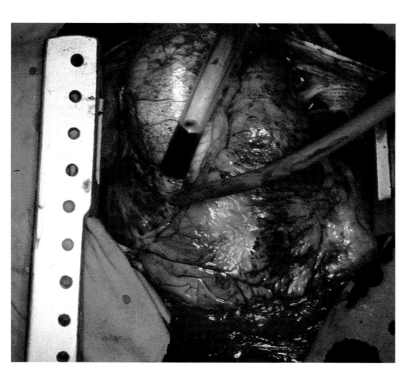

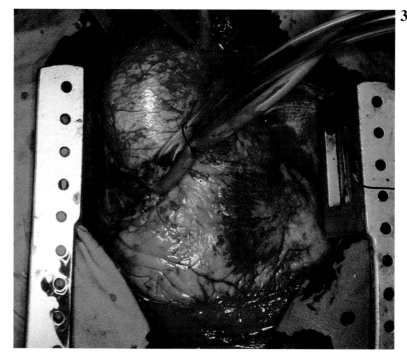

32

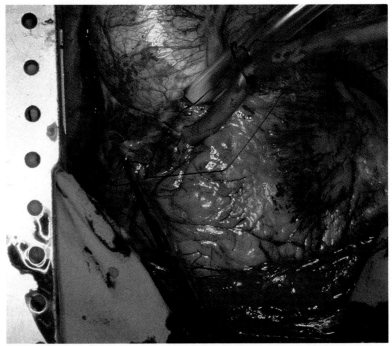

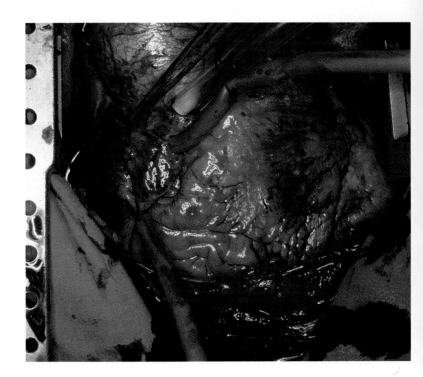

32 to 35 In this patient a second tube is to be inserted and therefore a diamond-shaped purse-string suture is inserted in the wall of the right atrium. It is important not to place this suture too close to the superior vena cava, as the sino-atrial node might be damaged. The suture is placed on a rubber snugger and the suture held up while an incision is made with a knife and the cannula inserted. The rubber is then snugged.

34

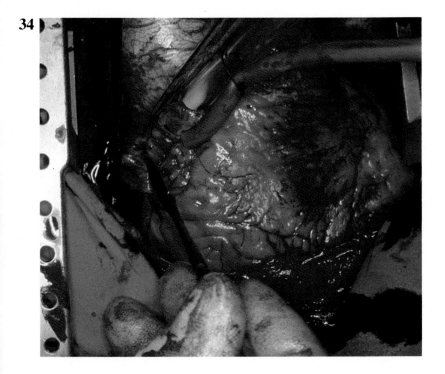

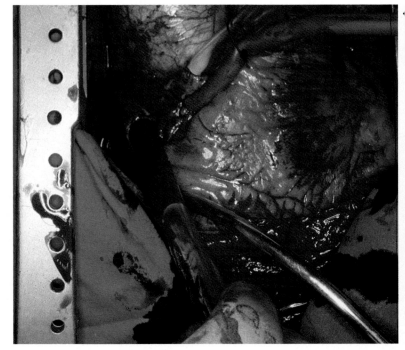

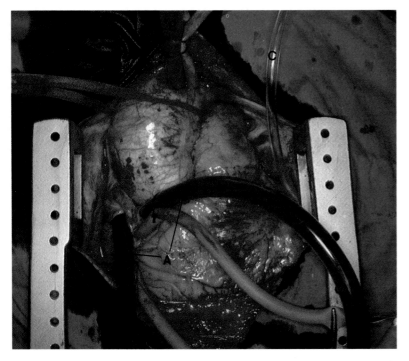

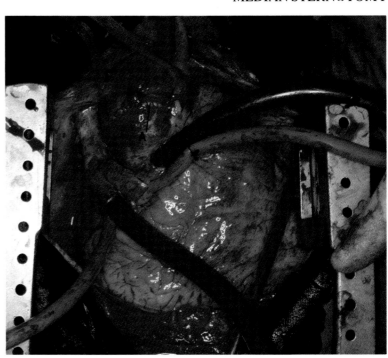

36   The second venous cannula is positioned in the superior vena cava and it is tied to the rubber snugger. This overall view shows the venous cannulae containing very desaturated blood (**A**), and the aortic cannula (**B**) containing saturated blood returning from the cardiopulmonary bypass machine as bypass has now been commenced. A tube (**C**) is in position to fill the pericardial space with cold fluid once the aorta is clamped and cardioplegic solution has been inserted.

37   The operation has been completed (in this case aortic and mitral valve replacement) and the aortic suture line is clearly seen (**A**). The venous cannulae can now be removed, and the stitch holding the superior vena cava cannula to the snugger has been cut.

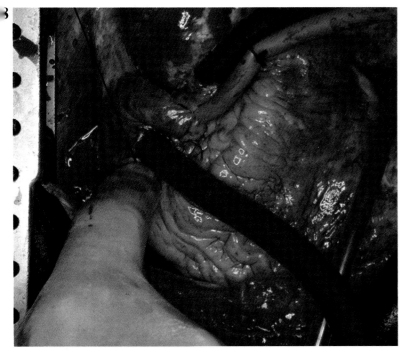

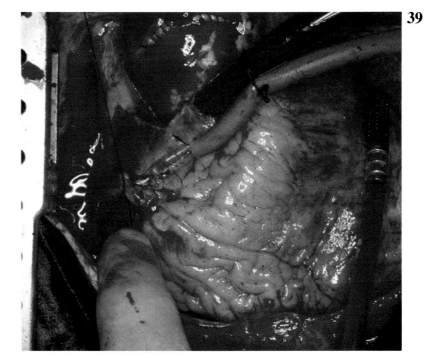

38 and 39   The rubber snugger is removed from the purse-string stitch, which is then tied down as the cannula is removed. An extra suture is then inserted to secure the cannulation site.

40

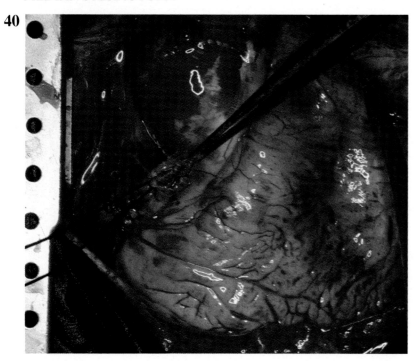

40 The other venous cannula has been removed from the right atrial appendage, which is doubly ligated.

41 to 43 Once all the blood needed has been returned to the patient from the cardiopulmonary bypass machine, the aortic cannula can be removed. The stitches holding it to the rubber snugger are cut and the purse-string suture tied as the cannula is removed. A Prolene suture is then inserted to secure the cannulation site and it is important that this stitch catches the media of the aorta, as otherwise a dissection might possibly occur.

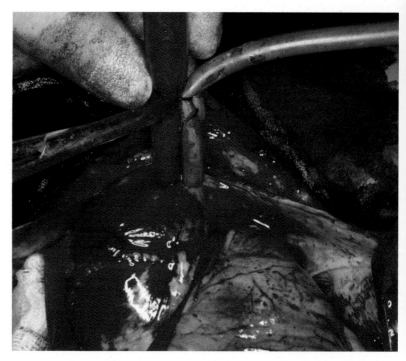

42

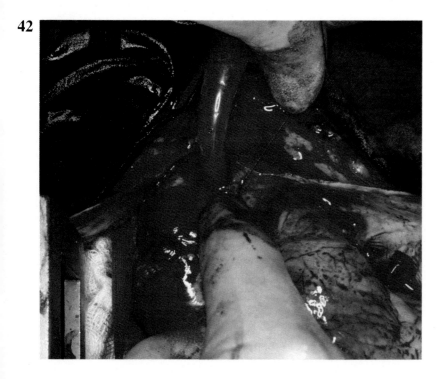

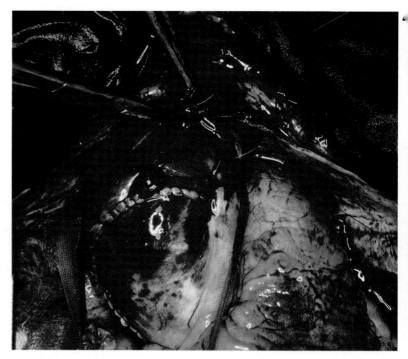

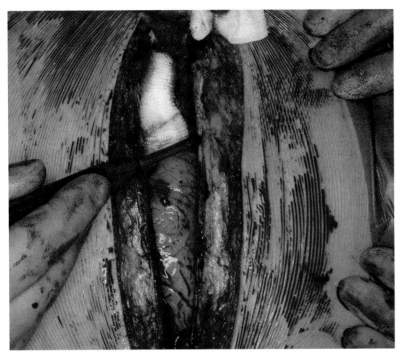

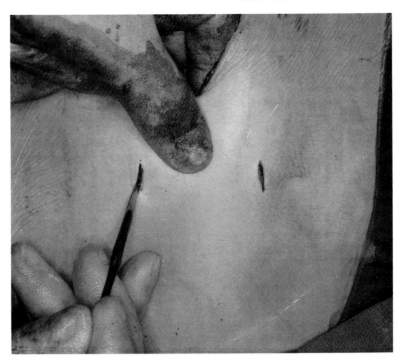

44 The sternal retractor and side-towels are removed and the sternal edges again diathermied and haemostasis generally secured.

45 to 47 Two drainage tubes are usually inserted to be connected to underwater seal drainage bottles on gentle suction. Two small skin incisions are first made and a suture inserted for tying later when the drain is removed. The tubes are then pulled through into position with Robert's forceps.

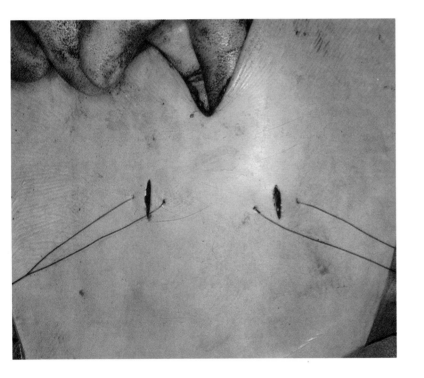

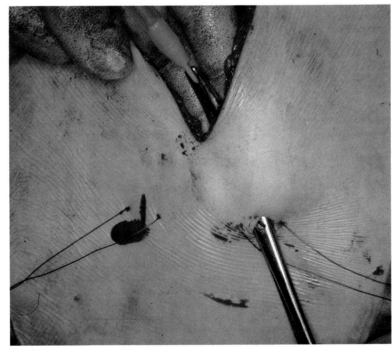

48

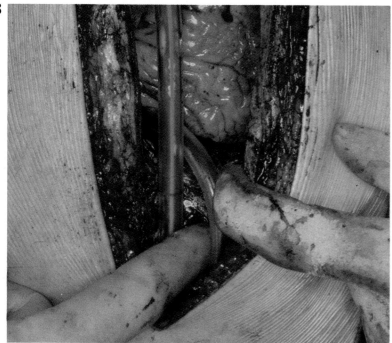

49

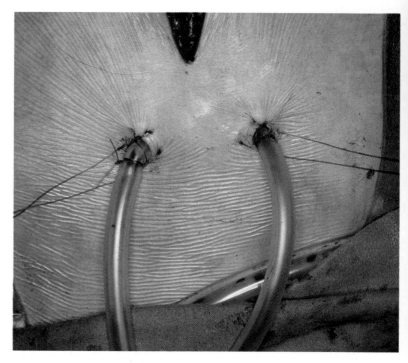

48 One tube is usually placed in front of the heart and one behind. However, if a graft has been performed to the right coronary artery, it is unwise to place a tube posteriorly as it might cause bleeding from the anastomosis.

49 The tubes are securely fixed in position with another suture.

50

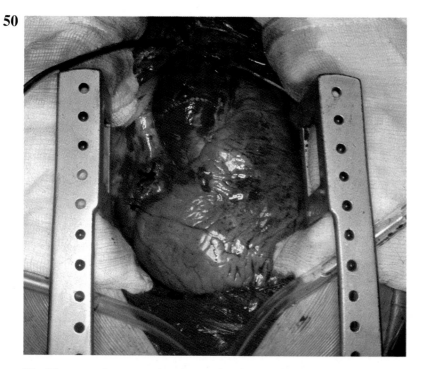

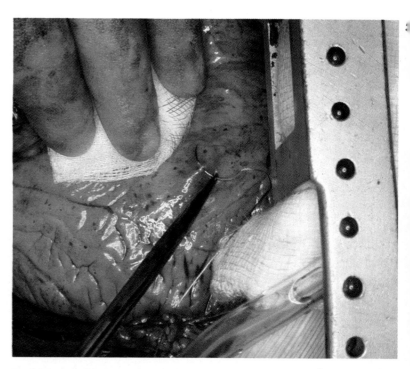

50 The sternal retractor is reinserted and a careful check made for any bleeding.

51 A temporary pacing wire is sutured carefully into the surface of the right ventricle. This is in case pacing is needed to increase the heart rate in the post-operative period. This suture is easily pulled out, usually on the 10th post-operative day.

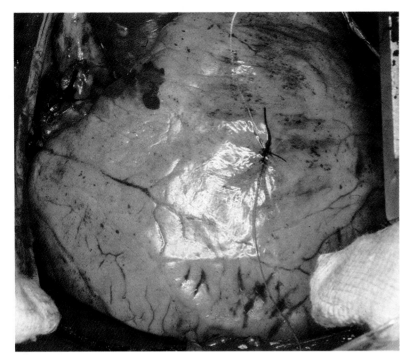

52   The pacing suture is secured in position with a stitch.

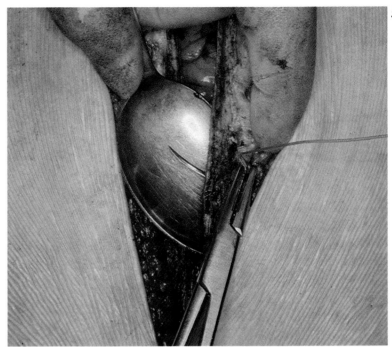

53 to 55   The sternum is approximated with a series of heavy, non-absorbable sutures. A spoon is helpful to protect the heart from the needle as it is placed through the sternum. The other sutures are crossed and pulled tight as the first knot is tied.

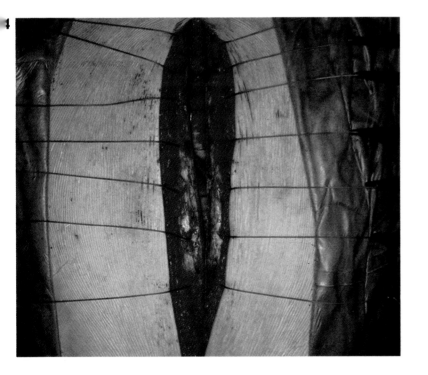

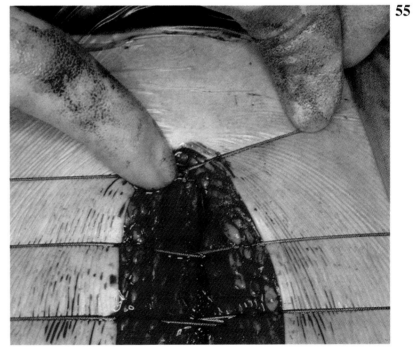

56

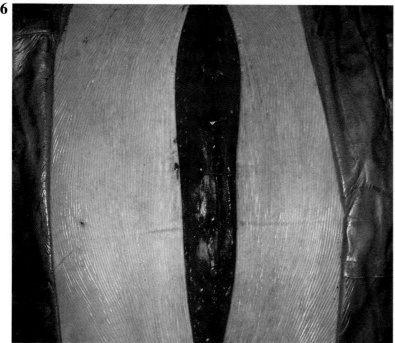

56 All the sternal sutures are tied securely. Some surgeons use wire to suture the sternum; there seems to be little difference. However, whichever method is used, the knots must be tight or there is a considerable risk of sternal dehiscence.

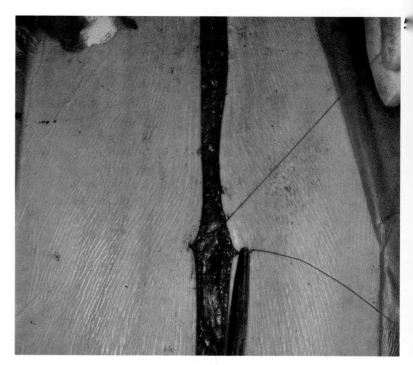

57 The periosteum and deep tissues are closed with continuous nylon. It is important to obliterate any deep space; otherwise leakage from the wound may occur post-operatively. Care must also be taken to approximate the rectus sheath inferiorly or the patient may subsequently develop an epigastric hernia.

58

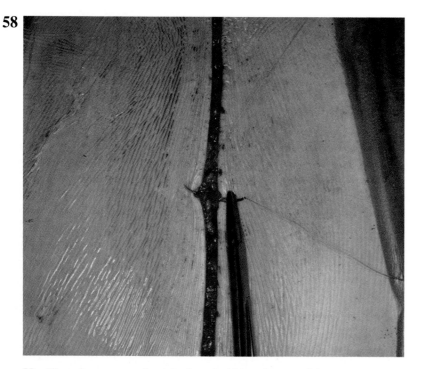

58 The subcutaneous tissue is closed with continuous plain catgut.

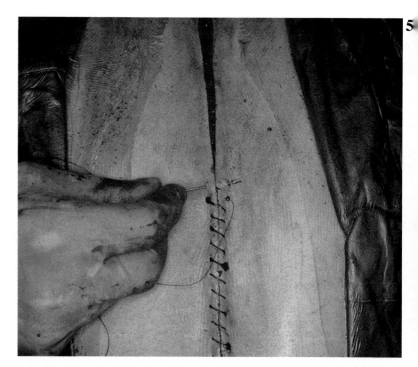

59 The skin is here closed with continuous nylon, but other methods such as subcuticular Dexon are equally satisfactory.

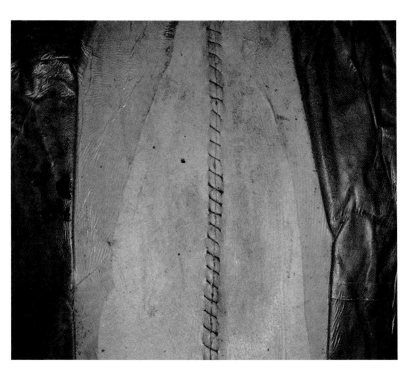 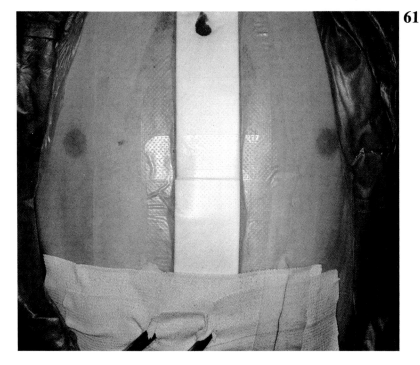

60 and 61 The finished wound is then covered with suitable dressings.

3: Thoracotomy

This is not a common approach in cardiac surgery, though obviously routine for thoracic surgery. A left thoracotomy is used in operations for coarctation of the aorta or resection of aneurysm of the descending aorta. Closed mitral valvotomy can be performed through this incision or, better, through a smaller and more anterior incision. It is also possible to perform mitral valve surgery and to close atrial septal defects through a right antero-lateral thoracotomy.

For repair of coarctation of the aorta it is usual to go through the fourth left intercostal space, but for aortic aneurysms it may be necessary to go through a lower space, depending on the site of the aneurysm.

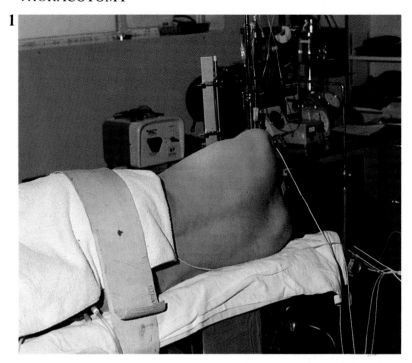

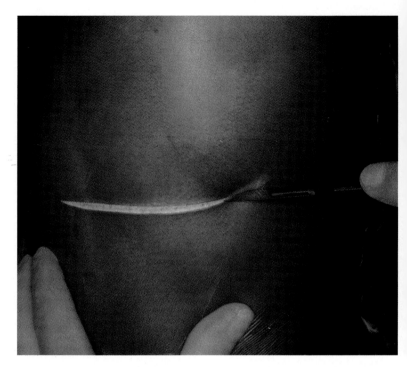

1   The patient is positioned on the operating table with the side of the chest to be operated on uppermost. The patient is firmly fixed with a strong strap over the hips. The skin is then sterilised and suitably draped.

2   The skin is incised with the knife but the incision is not carried deeper than 2–3 mm. The incision starts well below the nipple and runs posteriorly about 8 cm below the scapula and upwards, stopping well short of the midline.

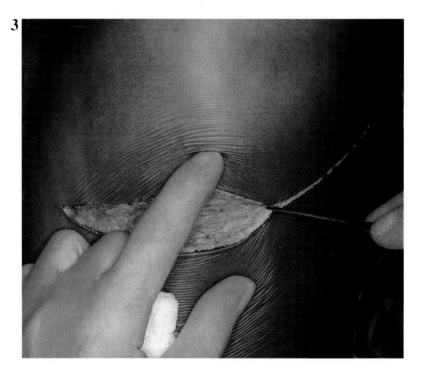

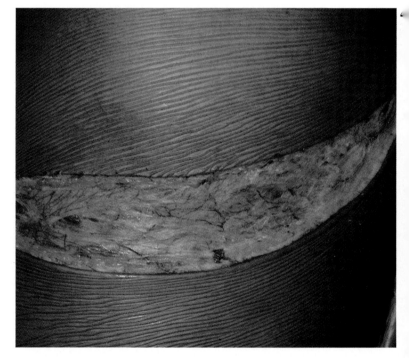

3 and 4   The subcutaneous fat is then incised with a diathermy to minimise bleeding.

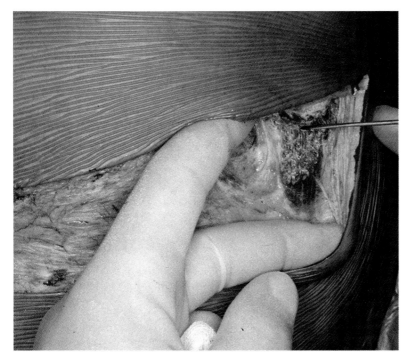

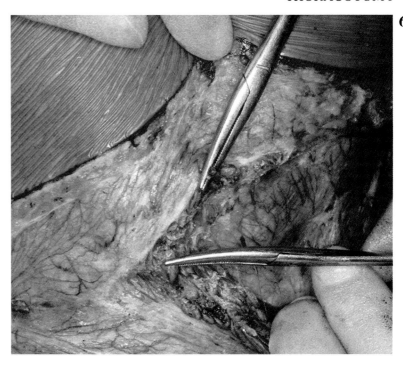

5 It is usually necessary to incise a short distance into the trapezius muscle.

6 The incision is carried forward through the more superficial latissimus dorsi and the deeper serratus anterior muscles. In this case, the patient has a coarctation of the aorta, and large intramuscular collateral arteries are being clamped.

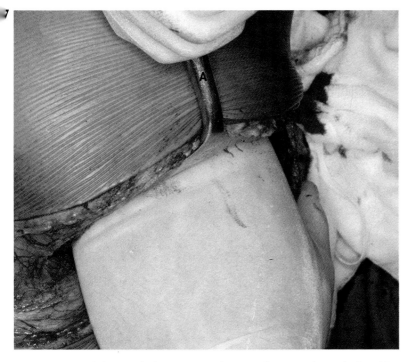

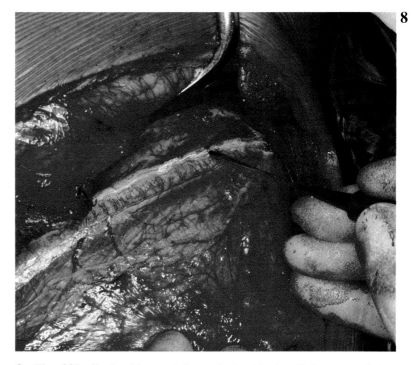

7 A retractor is inserted (**A**) to retract the scapula upwards, and a hand is inserted to feel the second rib and then count down to identify the fifth rib.

8 The fifth rib (in this case) is marked with the diathermy and the periosteum over the rib is incised with diathermy.

9

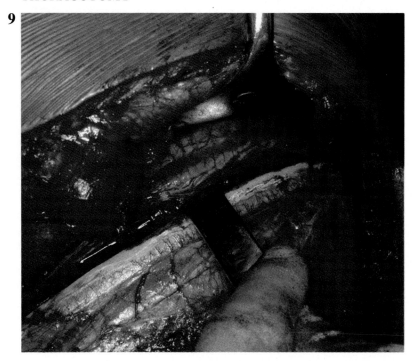

9 A periosteal elevator is then used to scrape the periosteum off the rib for the full length of the incision. Because of the line of attachment of the intercostal muscles, this is best done starting posteriorly and sweeping forward on the upper surface of the rib.

10

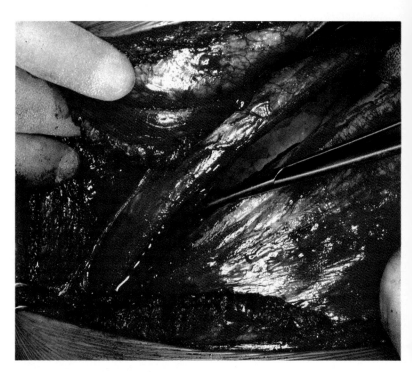

10 The pleura lying deep to the intercostal muscles, is then incised with scissors, releasing air into the pleural cavity.

11

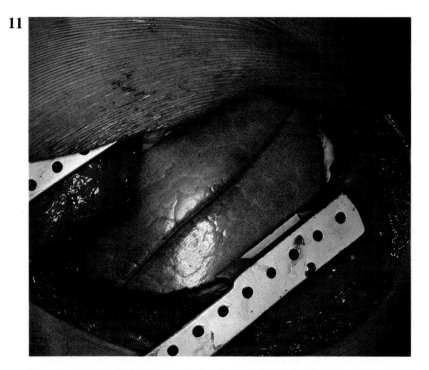

11 A self-retaining retractor is then inserted and the ribs spread apart to reveal the lung. The lung is retracted and the operation is performed.

12

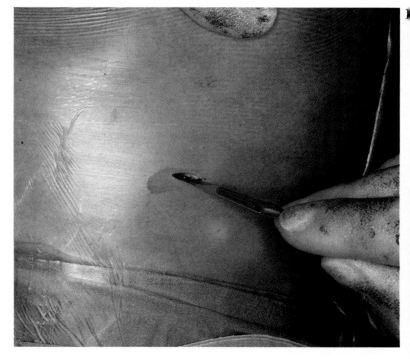

12 Once the operation has been performed, it is usual to insert a chest drain. A knife is used to make a hole several intercostal spaces below the incision.

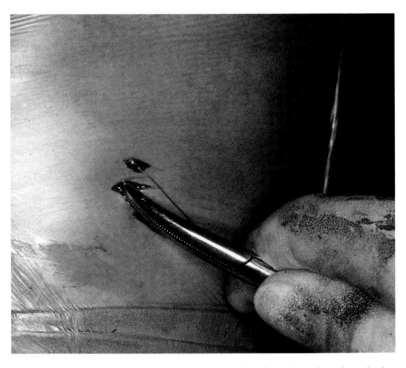

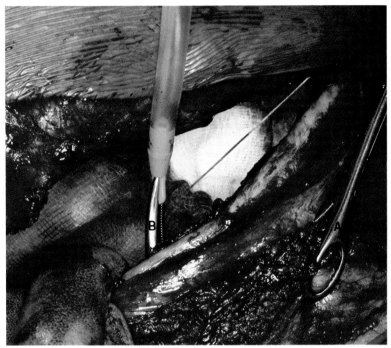

13 A stitch is placed loosely across the incision for tying when the tube is removed.

14 The muscles are held up with Lane's forceps (**A**) while Robert's forceps (**B**), which have been introduced into the chest through the little skin incision, are used to grasp the chest tube which is then pulled out through the skin.

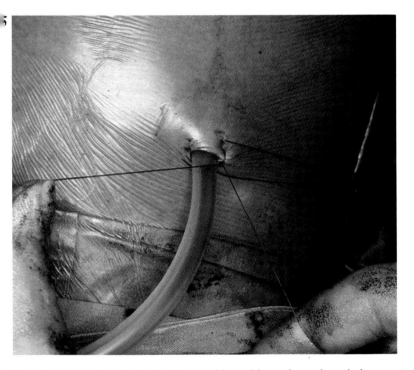

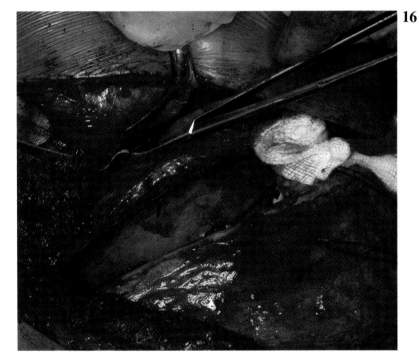

16

15 The tube is then firmly tied into position with another nylon stitch.

16 Two heavy chromic catgut pericostal sutures are then inserted to approximate the ribs. Care must be taken not to stab the lung.

17

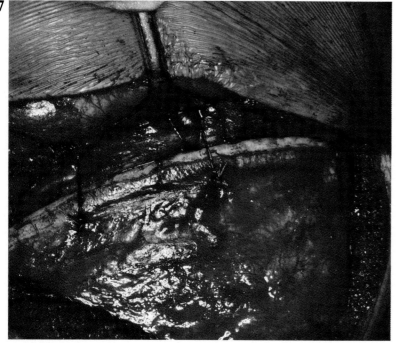

17 These two sutures are tied around the ribs. Some surgeons prefer to place sutures through the lower rib rather than around it, thus avoiding pinching the intercostal nerve.

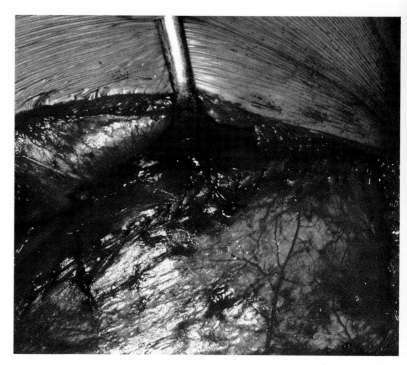

18 The intercostal muscle is then sutured over the rib below the continuous chromic catgut sutures.

19

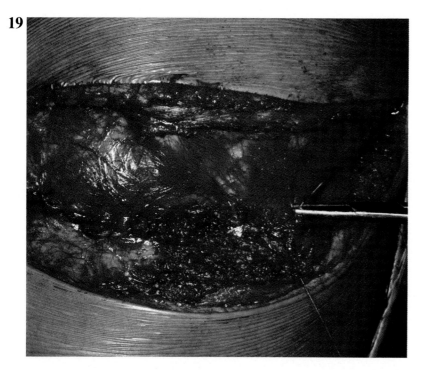

19 Starting anteriorly, the serratus anterior muscle is closed with continuous chromic catgut.

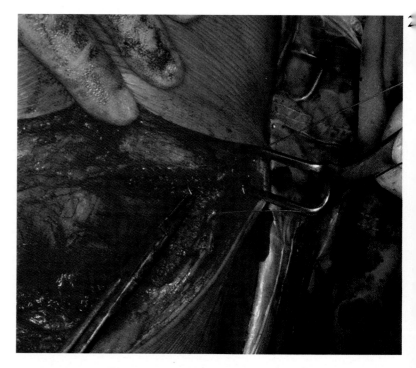

20 Starting posteriorly, the trapezius and latissimus dorsi muscles are closed with a second layer of chromic catgut.

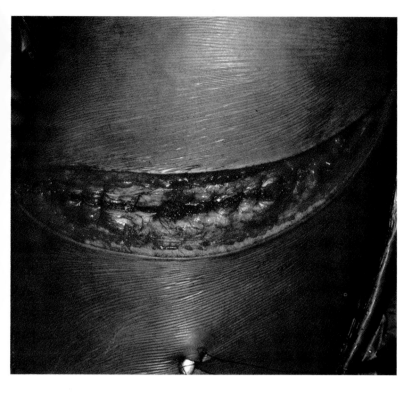

21 The latissimus dorsi muscle is shown resutured, and the subcutaneous layer is then closed with plain catgut.

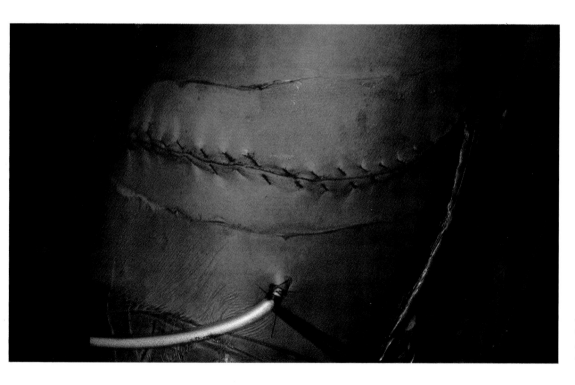

22 The skin is closed, in this case with continuous nylon, and the drainage tube can be seen emerging well below the wound.

4: Aortic valve replacement

Aortic valve disease remains one of the commonest and most eminently treatable conditions presenting to the cardiac surgeon. Rheumatic fever can cause aortic valve stenosis, and congenitally bicuspid valves usually narrow over the years. Both may result in heavily calcified, rigid valves and it may be impossible to determine the cause of stenosis. Aortic regurgitation may result from the rheumatic process, follow endocarditis or many other conditions. However, whether stenosed or regurgitant, there is virtually no place for repair of the aortic valve in adults, and valve replacement must be performed.

Harken[1] performed the first successful orthotopic valve replacement in 1960 and, since then, many different types of prosthetic valves have been used. Unfortunately, all the prosthetic valves tend to form thrombi on them and therefore patients must be anticoagulated. In the early 1960s ball valves, like the Starr–Edwards valve,[2] were the most commonly used, but in the last decade the disc valve, like the Bjork–Shiley valve,[3] seems to have become more popular.

Because of the disadvantage of having to use anticoagulants, Ross[4] and Barratt-Boyes[5] used human aortic valves (homografts). The technique of insertion is rather more difficult and time-consuming but the results with homograft valves sterilised in antibiotics have been very gratifying without the use of anticoagulants.[6] In order to overcome the difficulty of insertion and availability of homografts, pig valves mounted on frames were introduced and in the 1970s these valves became increasingly popular. They are slightly more thrombogenic than the homograft, but do not need anticoagulation after the first two months. Although their durability will not be so good as prosthetic valves, they are very useful, particularly in patients in whom anticoagulants are contra-indicated. Other tissues, such as heterograft pericardium and dura mater have also been used, but the large number of prosthetic and tissue valves available just emphasises that none is perfect, and different surgeons have their own valve preference.

Aortic valve replacement is carried out through a midline sternotomy and cardiopulmonary bypass is necessary. The right side of the heart is not opened and therefore one venous cannula is sufficient. As the aortic root is opened, no blood will be flowing down the coronary arteries and some method of myocardial preservation is needed. This can be achieved either by coronary perfusion with two tiny cannulae connected to the bypass circuit and with the heart beating, or more usually now with cardioplegia (see Chapter 1). If there is no aortic regurgitation, the cardioplegic solution can be infused through the aortic root; but if there is aortic regurgitation, the coronaries must be perfused directly.

Aortic valve replacement with Starr–Edwards valve

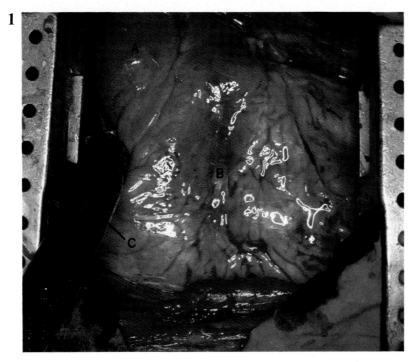

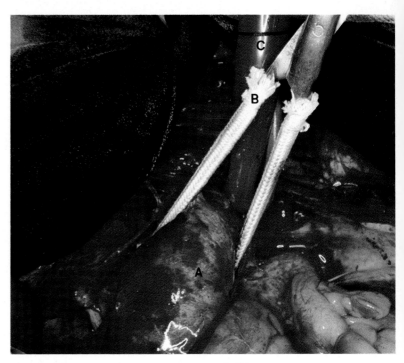

1 The overall view of the heart shows the aorta (**A**), right ventricle (**B**) and the single venous cannula (**C**) in the right atrial appendage.

2 Cardiopulmonary bypass has now been established, and the aorta (**A**) is about to be clamped with a cloth-covered cross-clamp (**B**). The aortic cannula (**C**) can be seen entering the aorta distal to the clamp.

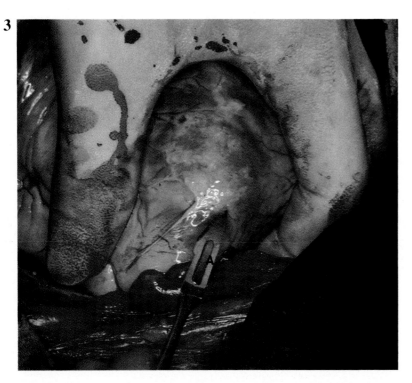

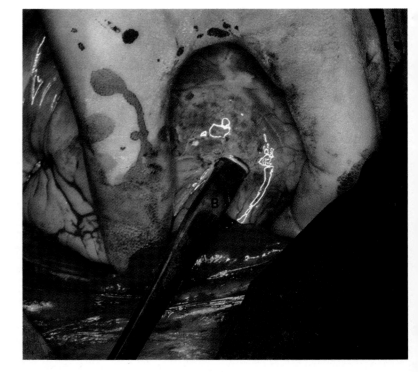

3 and 4 The heart is upended with the left hand and a small hole made to accept the left ventricular vent. The hole is initially made with a fine knife (**A**) and then enlarged with a pair of Robert's forceps (**B**).

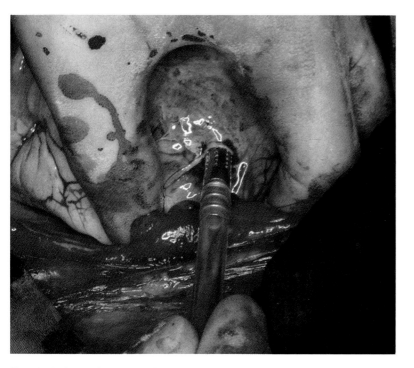

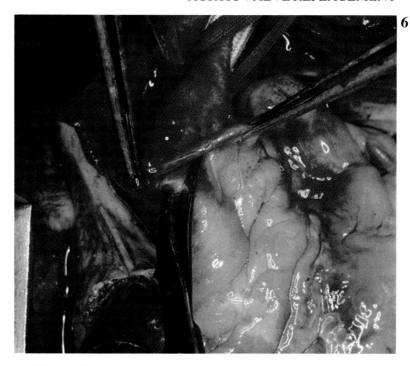

5 The left ventricular vent is then inserted and turned on gently.

6 The aorta is held with forceps so that the ascending aorta can be opened with scissors.

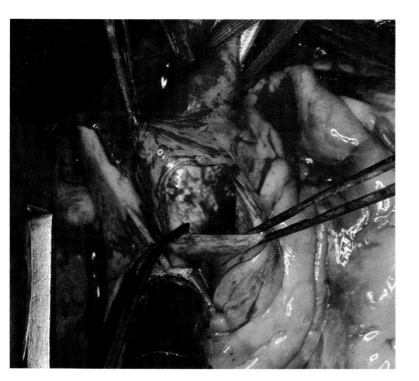

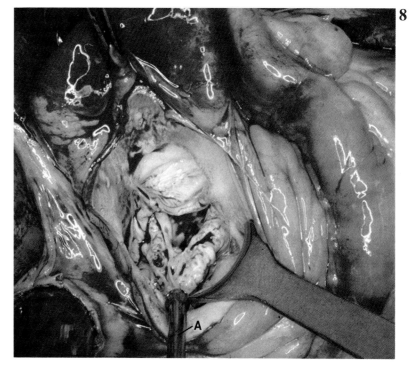

7 and 8 The aortic incision is extended down into the left coronary sinus and retraction reveals the heavily calcified valve. A sucker (**A**) points to the fused commissure between the right and non-coronary cusps.

9

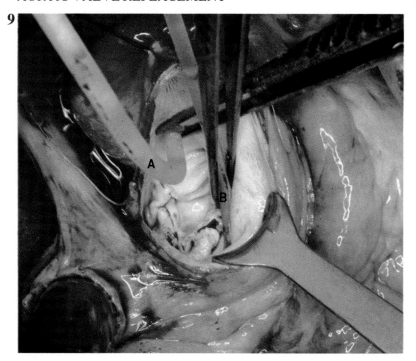

9 Cannulae have been inserted into the left (**A**) and right (**B**) coronary orifices and cardioplegic solution run in.

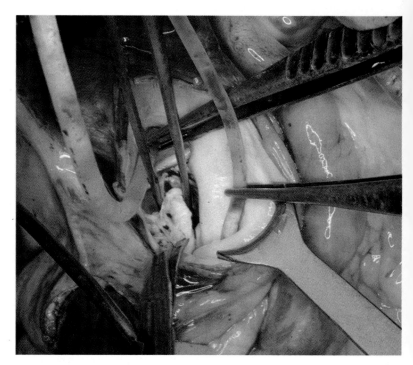

10 While the cardioplegic solution is infused, a start is made in excising the aortic valve.

11

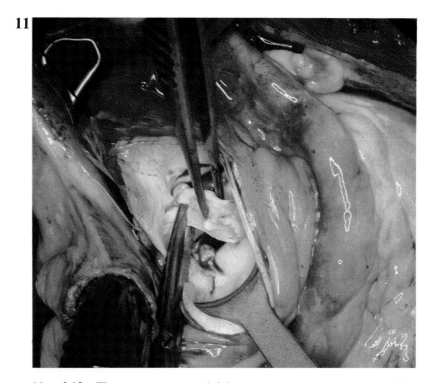

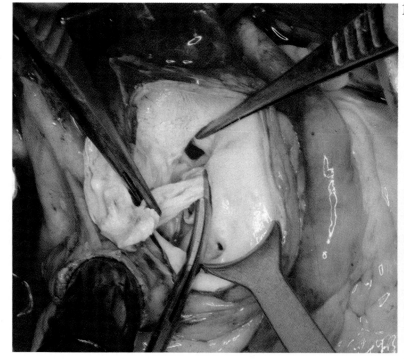

11 and 12 The non-coronary and right coronary cusps are removed with scissors, great care being taken to prevent any pieces of friable calcium from falling into the left ventricular cavity or left coronary artery.

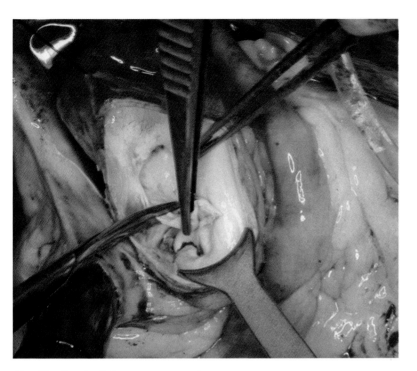

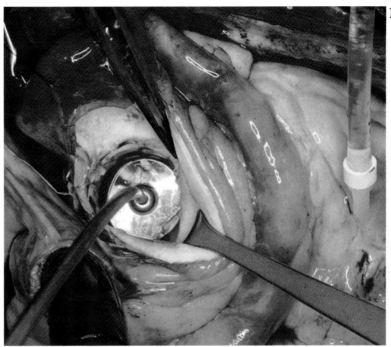

13 Finally, the left coronary cusp is removed. Any calcium in the valve ring must also be removed or the valve sutures might pull out.

14 Once the valve has been completely removed, the valve ring is measured to select the correct size of valve for replacement.

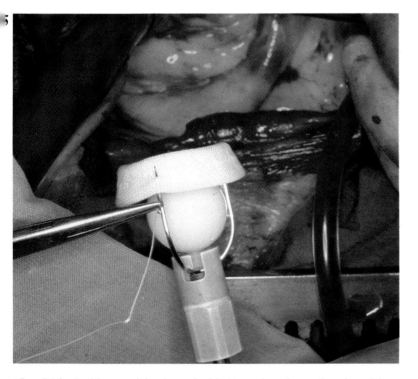

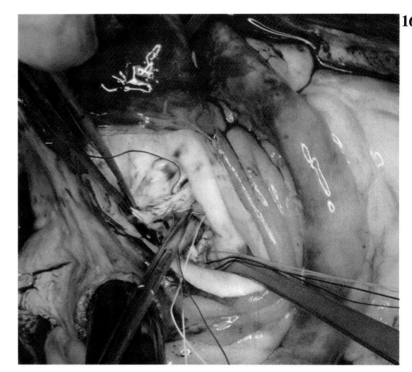

15 and 16 In this case, it has been decided to replace the aortic valve with a Starr–Edwards Model 1260 valve, which can be seen here held on its holder. Interrupted 2/0 sutures are placed first through the valve sewing ring and then into the aortic root. The sutures are inserted in a clockwise direction starting at the right end of the left coronary cusp remnant. It is helpful to use alternating sutures of different colours to make it easier to pick them up for tying.

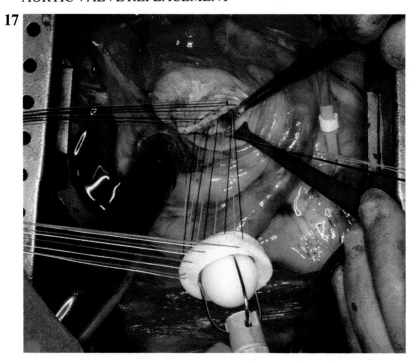

17 One third of the sutures have now been inserted into the left coronary cusp base and these sutures are clipped together and the needles cut off.

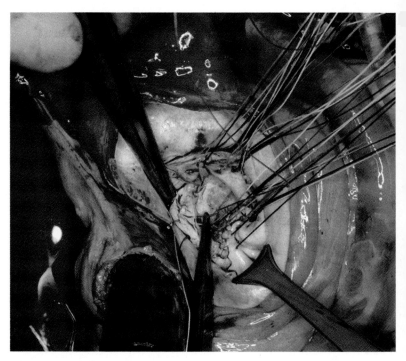

18 The sutures have been placed into the valve root at the base of the right coronary cusp and, continuing in a clockwise direction, a suture is being placed into the middle of the base of the non-coronary cusp.

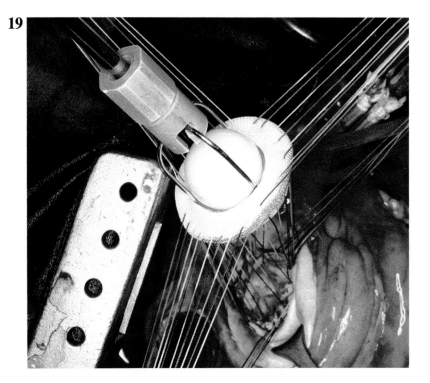

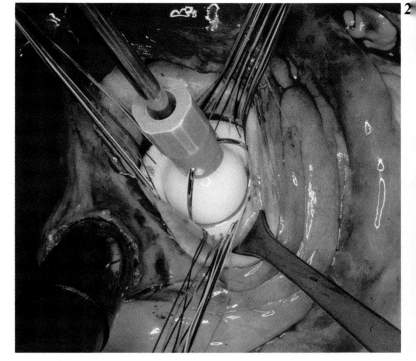

19 and 20 All the sutures are now in position and held in three groups so that the valve can be slid down into position and the valve holder removed leaving the valve in place.

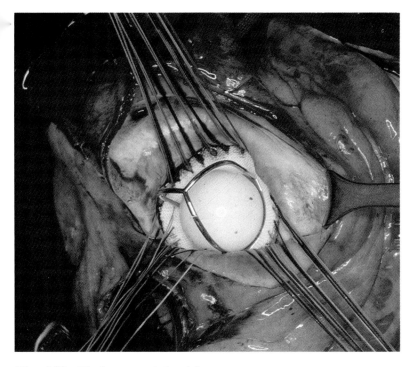
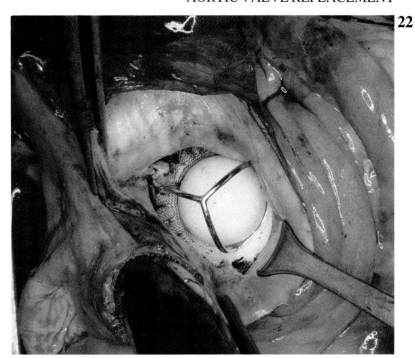

21 and 22 The knots are tied and the sutures are cut.

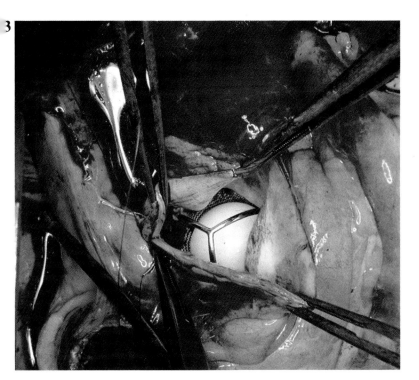
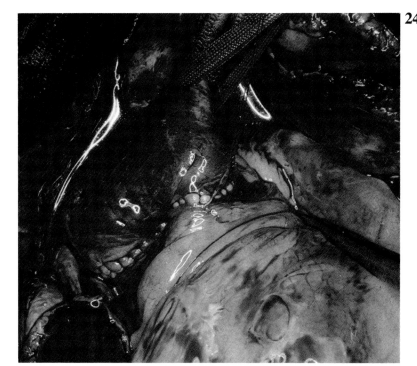

23 and 24 The aortic incision is closed with continuous 4/0 Prolene and, just before finally closing the suture line, the left ventricular vent is turned off, blood is returned to the patient and the anaesthetist ventilates the lungs, in order to remove all air from the heart.

25

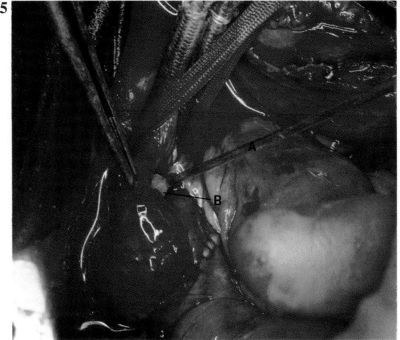

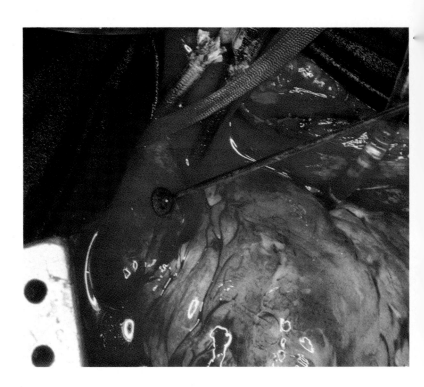

25 and 26 To safeguard further against any trapped air being released into the circulation, a needle (**A**) is placed in the ascending aorta. To prevent the needle slipping in too far, where it might either cause damage or miss any air, it has a flange (**B**) about 5 mm from the tip. The aortic clamp is released.

27

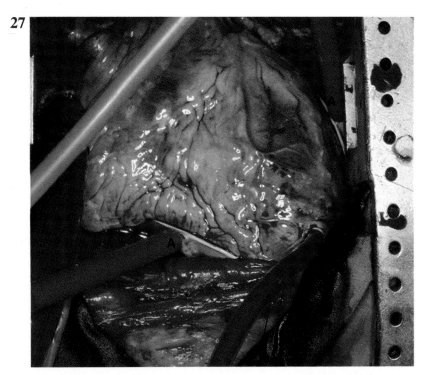

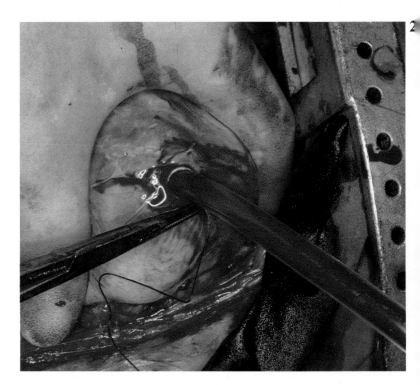

27 Frequently, the heart beats spontaneously once the aortic cross-clamp has been released and blood is flowing down the coronary arteries. However, ventricular fibrillation may develop, as in this case, and the heart is again upended to give a shock. The defibrillator paddles (**A**) can be seen.

28 The left ventricular vent can then be removed after checking that no more air remains in the left ventricle. Here a mattress suture is being inserted to close the hole after removal of the vent.

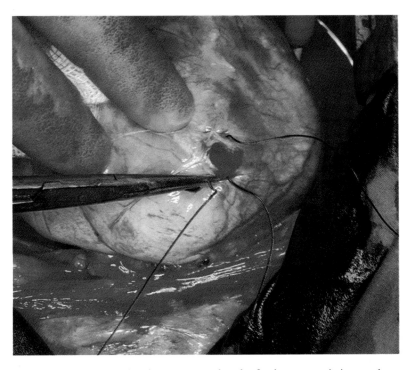

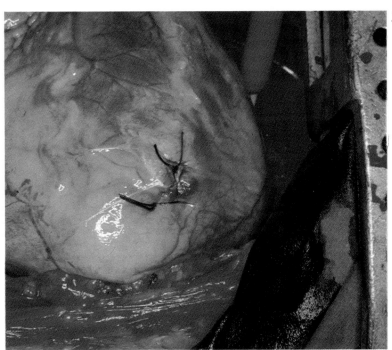

29 and 30 The vent has been removed and a further suture is inserted to ensure that the vent hole does not bleed.

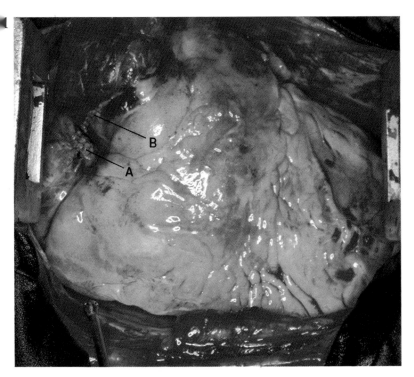

31 The heart is then replaced and once cardiopulmonary bypass has been discontinued the cannulae can be removed. The ligated right atrial appendage (**A**) has also been over-sewn after removal of the atrial cannula. The aortic suture line (**B**) is checked for bleeding.

Aortic valve replacement with Bjork–Shiley valve

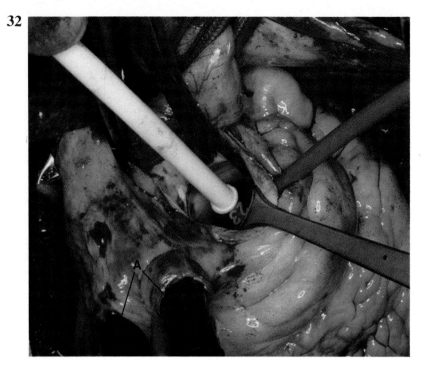

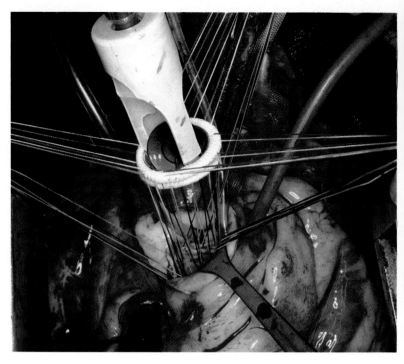

32 In this patient, it has been decided to replace the aortic valve with a Bjork–Shiley valve and, after excising the patient's valve, the valve ring size is being measured with a size 23 sizer. In this particular patient, the mitral valve was also replaced, so two venous cannulae (**A**) were used.

33 All the sutures have been inserted and the valve is ready to go down into the aortic root.

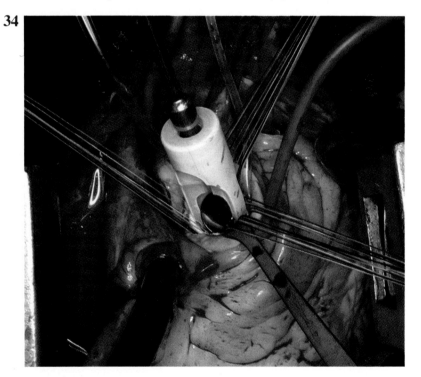

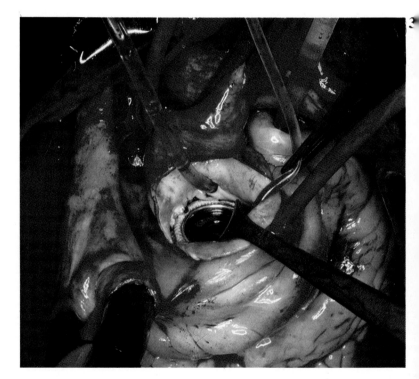

34 and 35 The valve is pushed down into position, the valve holder removed and the knots tied.

Aortic valve replacement with Carpentier–Edwards pig valve

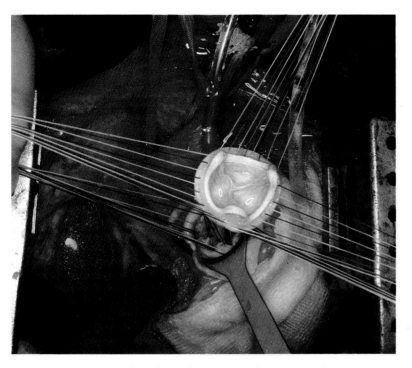

37

36 and 37 In this patient, it has been decided to insert a pig valve. The technique of insertion is similar to that for a prosthetic valve because the valve is mounted on a stent which has a sewing ring. All the sutures have been inserted and the valve is slid down into position.

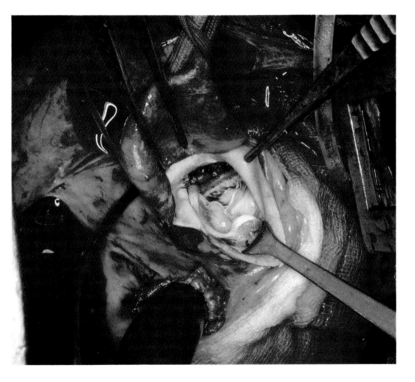

38 The knots have been tied and the three thin, glistening valve cusps can be seen.

Aortic valve replacement with a homograft valve

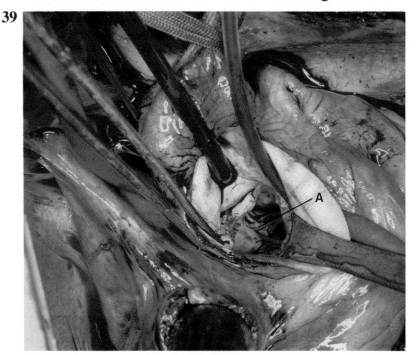

39   The aortic valve has been removed and, at this stage in this particular operation, coronary perfusion is being used and the heart is beating. The anterior leaflet of the mitral valve (**A**) can be clearly seen.

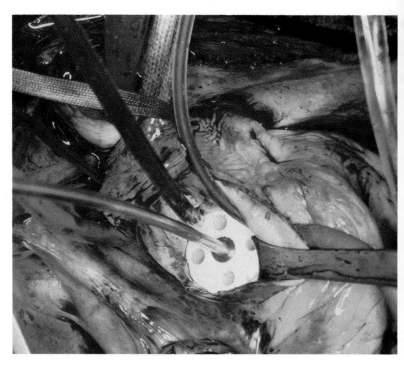

40   The size of the valve ring is measured and a homograft is selected with an internal diameter 2 mm less than the transverse diameter of the aortic root.

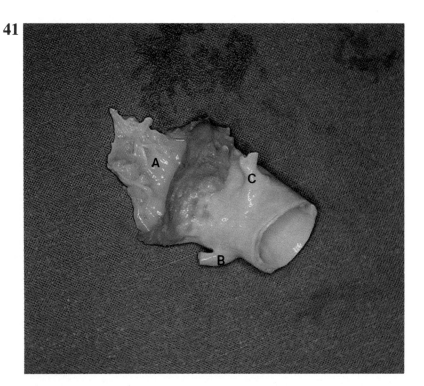

41   The aortic homograft containing the aortic valve has been sterilised in antibiotic solution,[6] and stored at 4°C. It is washed in saline prior to trimming. The anterior leaflet of the mitral valve (**A**), left coronary artery (**B**) and right coronary artery (**C**) can be seen.

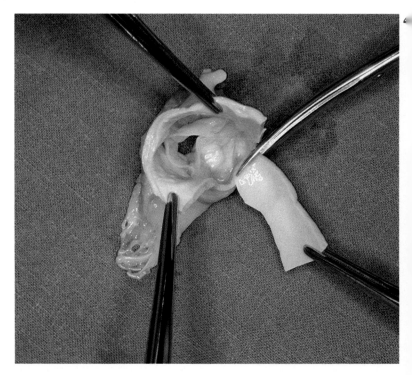

42   The valve is trimmed so as to remove the aortic wall in the sinuses of Valsalva, but leaving a strip of tissue for suturing adjacent to the cusp. Here, part of the aortic wall in the non-coronary sinus is being removed.

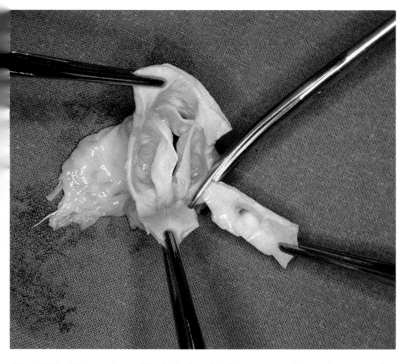

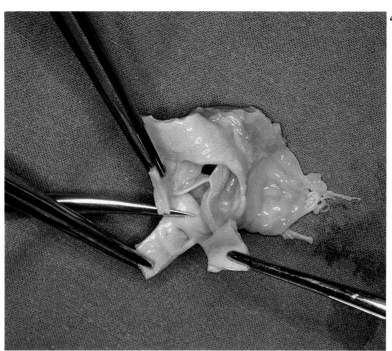

43 and 44 The aortic wall in the left and right coronary sinuses is removed.

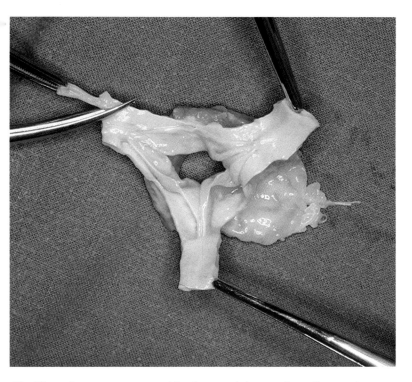

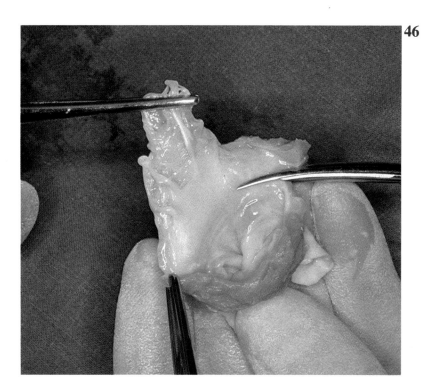

45 The valve cusps supported by the remaining aortic wall commissures are seen. The excess aortic wall is trimmed off.

46 The anterior leaflet of the mitral valve is removed, leaving a rim of tissue about 4 mm below the valve cusps.

47

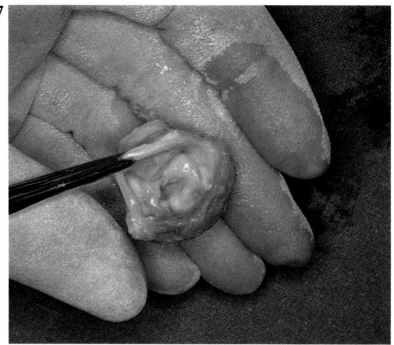

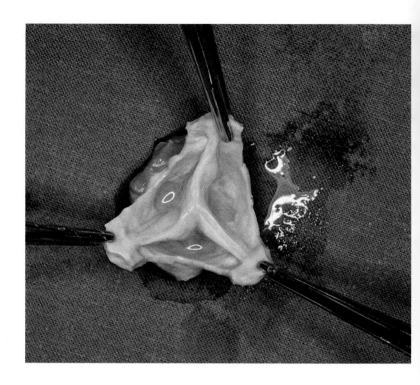

47 and 48 The final views from below and above show the valve ready for insertion.

49

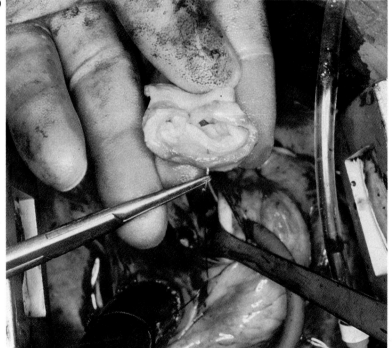

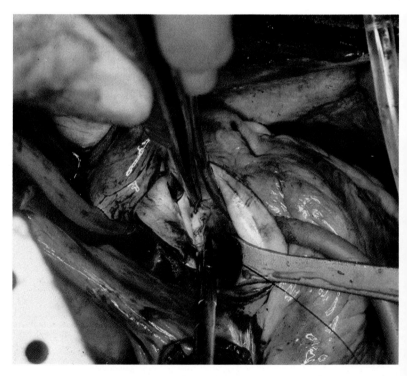

49 The insertion of the homograft now begins, and in this case cardioplegic solution has been infused down the coronary cannulae to facilitate insertion. The first 3/0 silk suture is inserted into the base of the homograft into muscle below the right coronary cusp.

50 The same suture is then inserted into the base of the patient's excised left coronary cusp. This results in a 120° anti-clockwise rotation of the homograft.

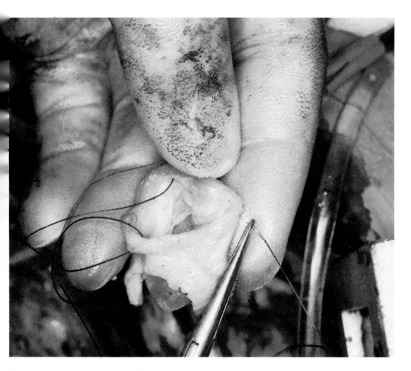

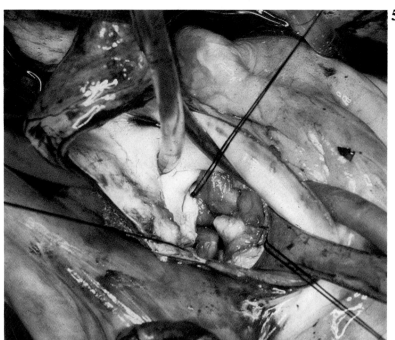

51 and 52 Two more silk sutures are placed through the homograft base and respective patient's cusp base, so that when the valve is slid down, the respective cusp bases can be tied together. Before doing this, the valve is turned inside out by pushing it through itself into the ventricle. The sutures are not cut, but left long for sewing in the base of the valve.

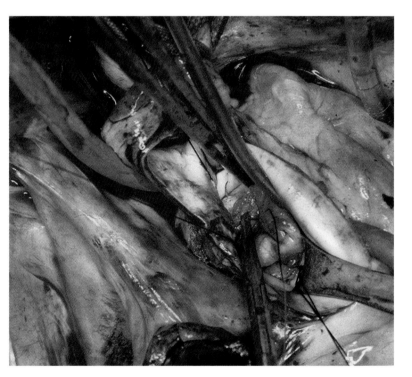

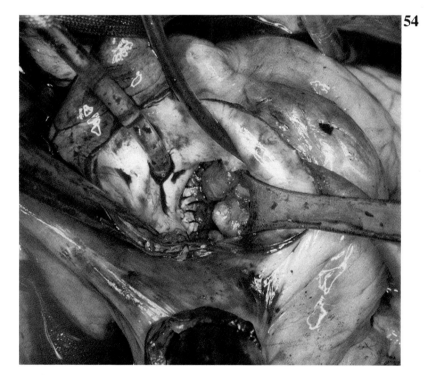

53 and 54 Starting with the suture tied to the base of the patient's left coronary cusp, the base is sutured in with continuous sutures in a clockwise direction, locking them at each cusp base.

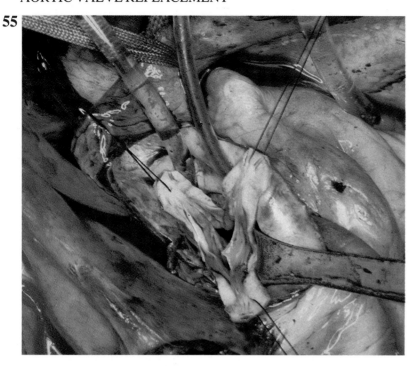

55 The valve is then carefully pulled back up the right way and a suture placed above each commissure.

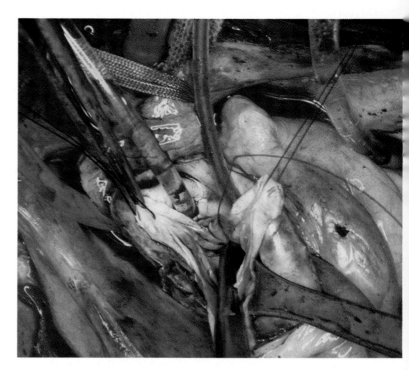

56 A suture is placed below each commissure into the aortic wall behind to hold the valve to the aortic wall. This has been found to reduce considerably the incidence of subsequent peripheral leaks.

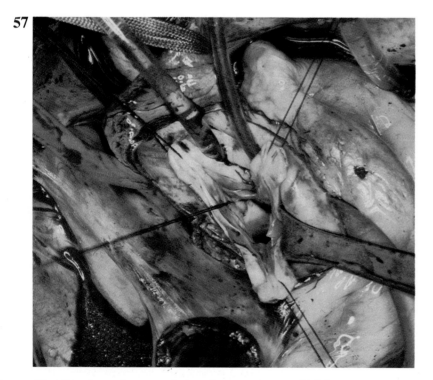

57 This shows the suture below the commissure which is now cut, care being taken not to damage the cusps.

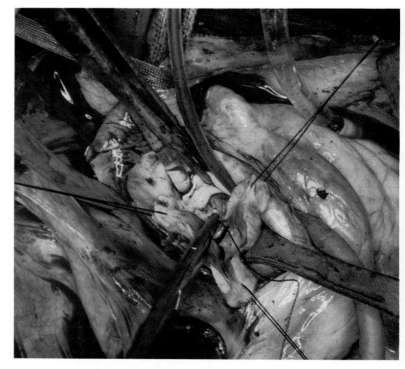

58 With a double-ended 3/0 silk, a suture is placed through the homograft above the base of the cusp and into the aorta well below the left coronary orifice. This suture is then tied and one end held.

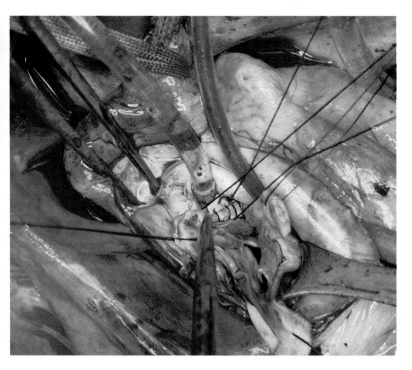

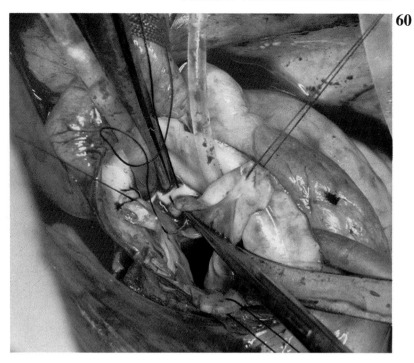

59   The other end is then used to run continuously up the edge of the aorta towards the commissure between the left and non-coronary cusps. This is then tied at the top to the suture already holding this commissure.

60   The other end of the same suture is then continued in the other direction taking care to stay well away from the left coronary orifice.

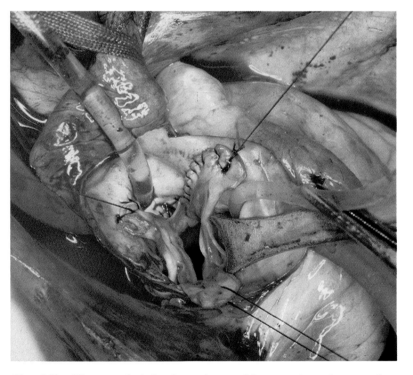

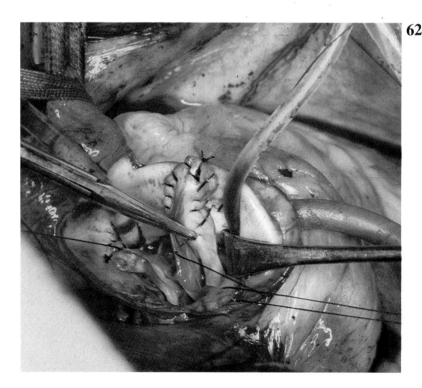

62

61 and 62   The suture is tied to that at the top of the commissure between the left and right cusps and this is then run around above the right coronary cusp taking care to avoid the right coronary artery.

63

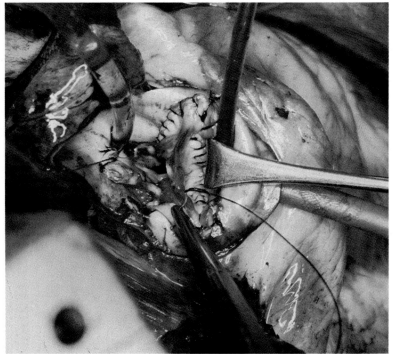 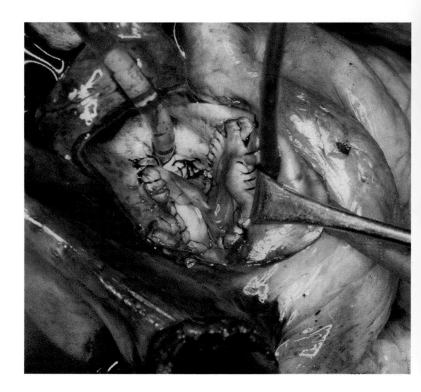

63 and 64   The final suture is carried around above the non-coronary cusp and tied. The final picture shows the valve cusps opposing; the coronary cannulae are then removed and the aorta is closed.

This technique is exactly that described by Barratt-Boyes[7] and it is obviously a much more difficult and precise operation than the insertion of a prosthetic valve. The homograft valve must be perfect, and the judging of the size of valve needed and the placement of the valve without damaging the delicate cusps require considerable experience. It is recommended that insertion of a homograft should only be attempted after considerable experience in a unit undertaking many such operations. Some surgeons use other suture materials and minor modifications of the technique.

5: Mitral valve repair

As long ago as 1923, Cutler[1] performed the first successful mitral valvotomy in Boston, USA. His approach was rather different from that used today, and if, as was his intention, he had made the valve incompetent, his patient might not have survived. It was not until the late 1940s that mitral valvotomy became an accepted surgical procedure, the heart being approached through a left thoracotomy. Initially the mitral valve was split with a finger through the left atrium only, but later with the use of the Tubbs dilator (see diagram **A**), a better split of the stenotic mitral valve could be achieved. However, this operation is performed with the heart beating and there is a risk that a clot in the left atrial appendage, or calcium from the valve, could embolise, causing serious cerebral problems. In addition, the valve could tear or be incompletely split. Nevertheless, a large number of these operations were performed and, with careful case selection,

very good results were achieved on the whole. However, most Western surgeons now prefer to perform mitral valvotomy on cardiopulmonary bypass so that the valve can be seen directly and the maximum relief of stenosis achieved. Furthermore, it is possible to test the valve for regurgitation and if more than trivial regurgitation is present, a Carpentier ring[2] can be inserted in an attempt to make the valve competent. If, however, this fails, the surgeon is in a much better position to replace the valve than if a 'closed' valvotomy had been performed.

For 'open' mitral valvotomy and repair, cardiopulmonary bypass is obviously used. Most surgeons approach the mitral valve through a median sternotomy, as shown in this chapter, but a right thoracotomy can also be used, although removal of air is not so easy with the latter approach.

Closed mitral valvotomy

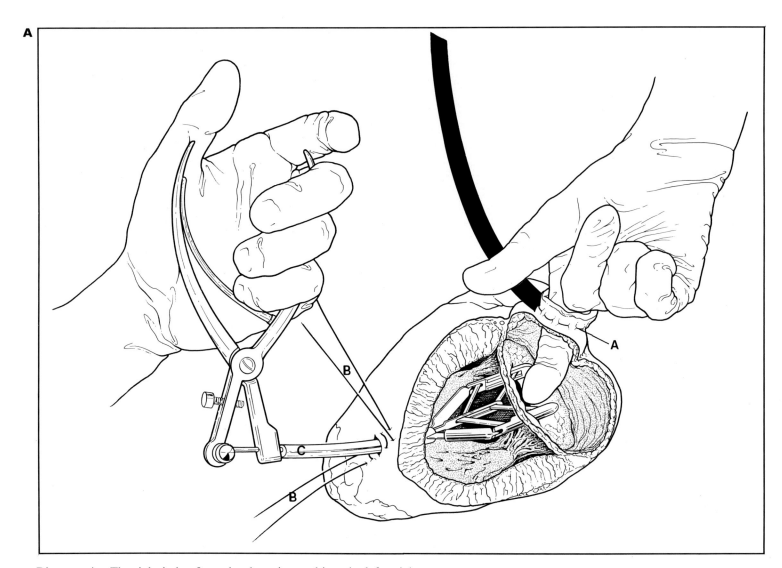

Diagram A   The right index finger has been inserted into the left atrial appendage and a purse-string suture (**A**) is snugged to prevent leakage of blood. Sutures (**B**) have been placed in the left ventricular apex, and the Tubbs dilator (**C**) inserted into the ventricle and guided retrogradely through the stenosed mitral orifice on to the tip of the finger in the left atrium. The valve is then quickly split by squeezing the handles of the Tubbs dilator, which opens the blades. The dilator should not be left in the stenosed mitral orifice for very long as, if the stenosis is really severe, this can virtually occlude the mitral orifice and cause the cardiac output to fall abruptly. Following the split, any regurgitation can be checked for with the finger, and the finger is removed and the appendage snugged. The dilator is then removed and the stay sutures tied. The left atrial appendage is then amputated or tied so that clot cannot collect in it.

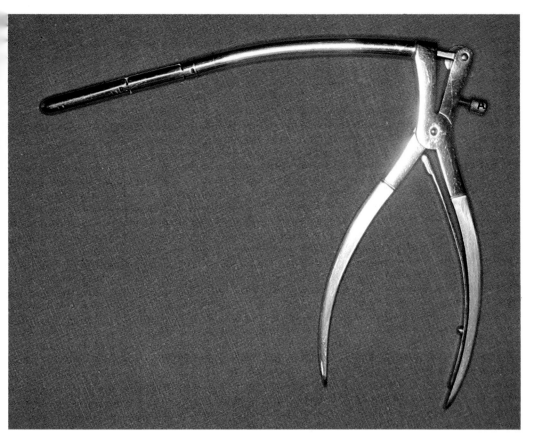

1 The Tubbs transventricular dilator is seen with the blades closed, the handle grip being held open by a spring. The screw (**A**) is used to adjust the distance which the blades will open, and this allows the surgeon to split the valve exactly however much he thinks is appropriate.

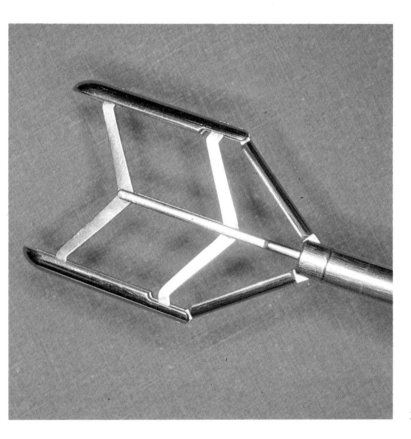

2 The blades of the Tubbs dilator have been opened to 4 cm.

Open mitral valvotomy

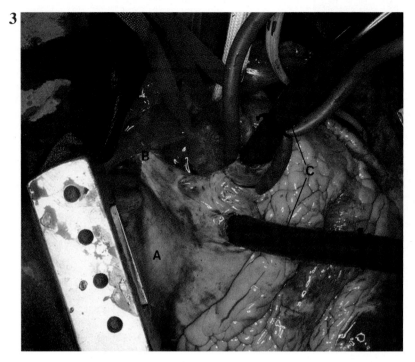

3 The rather inaccessible left atrium (**A**) is just seen behind the interatrial groove. The superior vena cava (**B**) and venous cannulae (**C**) can also be seen.

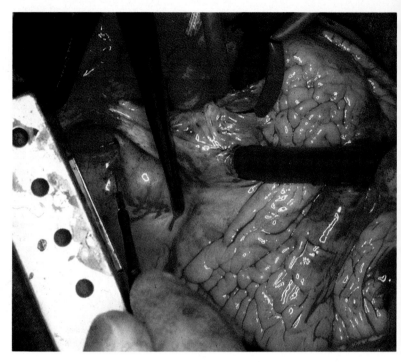

4 A vertical incision into the left atrium is made with a knife and then enlarged with scissors.

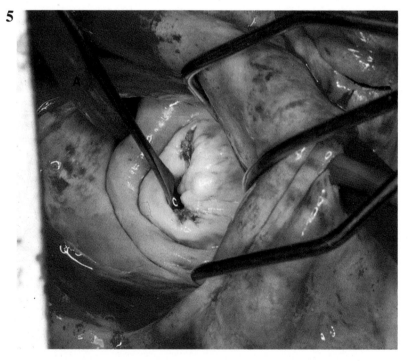

5 The heart is retracted to the left and the mitral valve exposed by retraction to the right, with a fine, long retractor which has been placed into the extremely stenosed orifice of the mitral valve. The diameter of the valve orifice in this case is less than 1 cm and the fused commissures contain some calcium. A sucker (**A**) returns blood to the bypass machine.

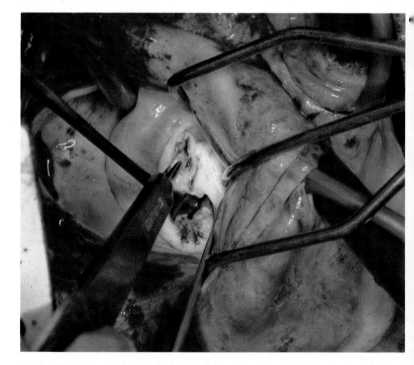

6 In this case, starting at the edge of the valve ring, the lateral commissure is divided carefully with a knife.

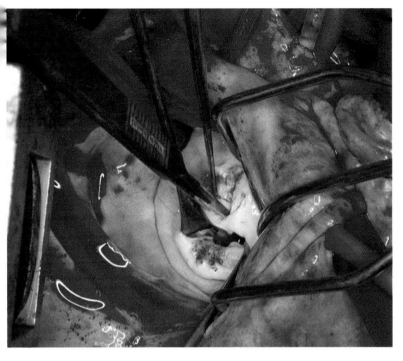
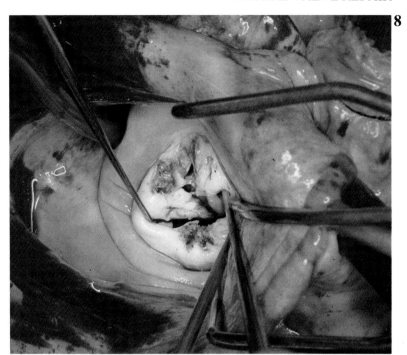

7 and 8   With the help of Blalock hooks, used to hold open the valve orifice, the division of the fused lateral commissure is completed.

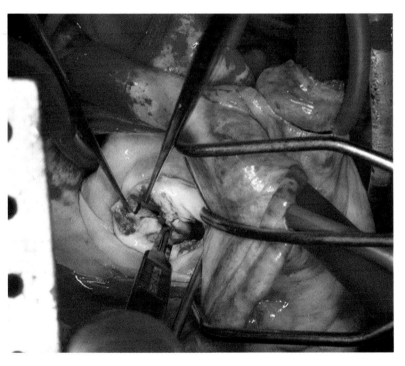
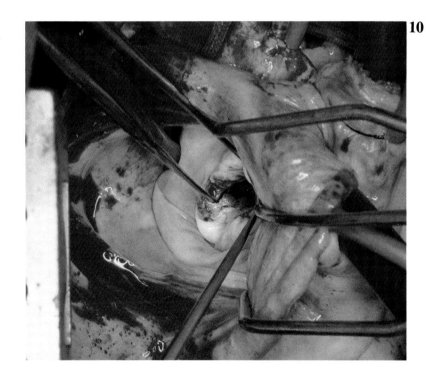

9 and 10   The fused papillary muscles and chordae are carefully divided downwards, to allow a wider orifice.

11

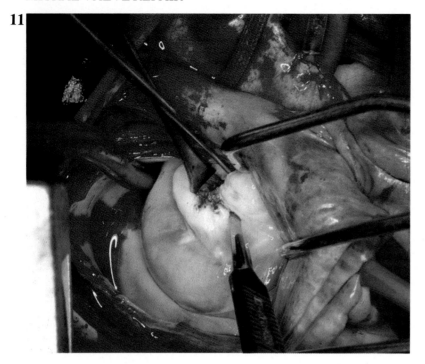

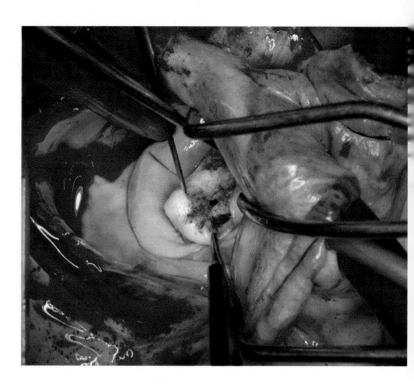

11 to 14 The medial commissure is now divided with the knife and the full relief of the stenosis of the valve is achieved.

13

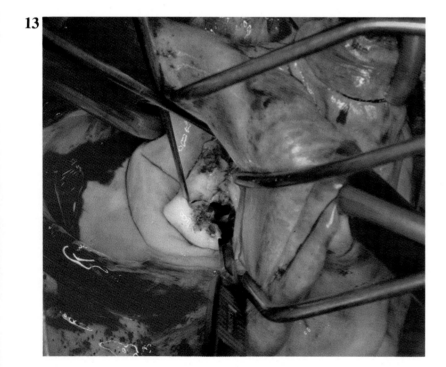

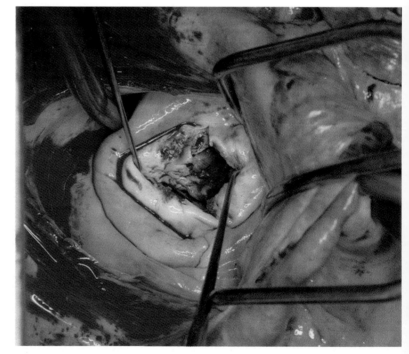

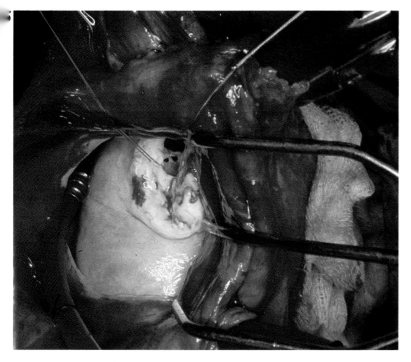

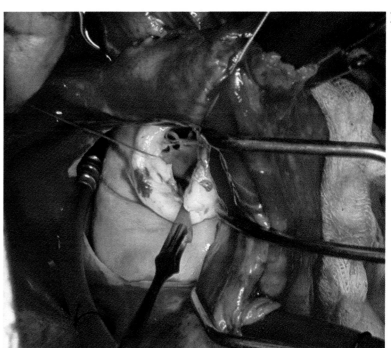

15 and 16 In a different patient, the anterior and posterior commissures have been held apart with stay sutures, and the medial commissure is being divided from within outwards.

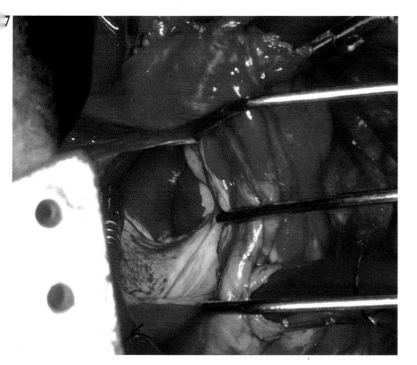

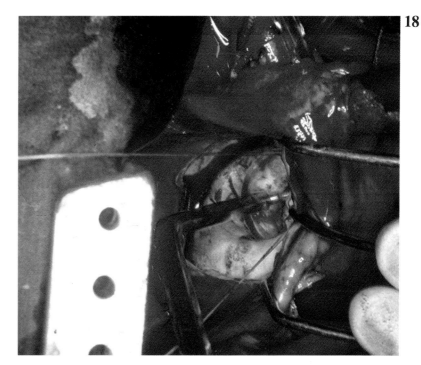

17 The valve is being tested by perfusing the aortic root with blood from the pump in order to let the heart beat. The left ventricle has been filled with blood through a vent and it can be seen that although the anterior leaflet is bulging back there is considerable central regurgitation.

18 It has been decided to insert a Carpentier ring and the valve is being measured for this.

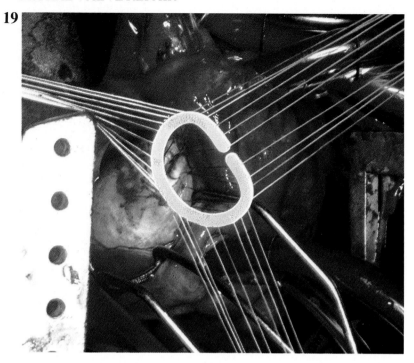

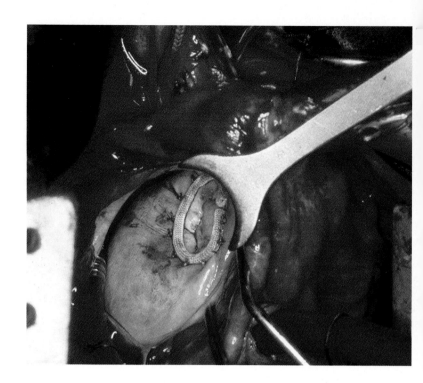

19 and 20 The Carpentier ring is inserted with interrupted sutures and tied into position, thus narrowing the mitral valve ring to the correct size and allowing the cusps to meet.

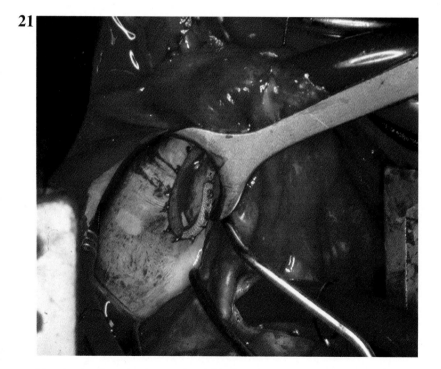

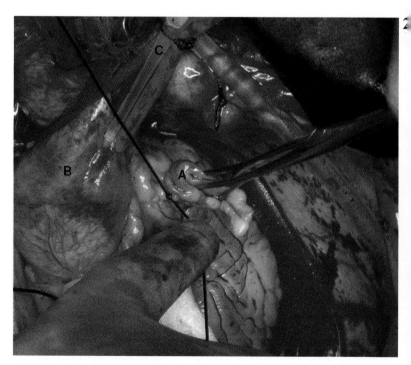

21 Again, the valve is tested and this time there is virtually no leak.

22 The left atrial appendage (**A**) is tied off to prevent thrombus formation in it. The appendage can also be occluded from inside by suturing off its orifice. The ascending aorta (**B**) still containing the cannula for insertion of the cardioplegic solution (**C**) is clearly seen.

6: Mitral valve replacement

The usual approach for this operation is through the midline, although some surgeons use the right chest approach, and it is possible to replace the mitral valve through the left chest. Obviously the operation must be performed with the use of cardiopulmonary bypass and, although it is possible to use only one venous cannula, it is usual to use two as the firm retraction necessary to see the mitral valve can occlude the cavae. Once cardiopulmonary bypass is established, the aorta is cross-clamped and cardioplegic fluid is infused into the ascending aorta (see Chapter 1). Direct incision into the left atrium with retraction gives a fair view of the mitral valve, particularly if there is a large left atrium. However, when the left atrium is small and if the left ventricle is stuck down by adhesions resulting from a previous operation, the view may be rather limited.

All the available valve substitutes are inferior to the human mitral valve and therefore valve replacement should only be undertaken when conservation is unsuitable. The valve may be replaced by one of the many prosthetic valves available such as the Bjork–Shiley valve[1] illustrated in this chapter, or by a tissue valve such as the stented glutaraldehyde-prepared pig valve.[2] There are also many different methods of suturing the valve in position. Either continuous or interrupted sutures may be used and the interrupted sutures may be single or mattress, with or without supporting pledgets of Teflon felt.

It is important to remove all air from the heart at the end of the procedure, and once the atrium is closed it is usual to tip up the left ventricle and vent the apex. The aorta is vented before release of the aortic clamp and this vent is not removed until bypass is stopped.

Following insertion of a prosthetic valve, anticoagulants will be used for the rest of the patient's life. Therefore, it may not be necessary to obliterate the left atrial appendage. However, when a tissue valve is inserted, even though anticoagulants are often used for the first two months or so post-operatively, particularly if the patient is in atrial fibrillation, there is a risk of clots forming in the appendage and it should be obliterated. This can be done either by suturing it closed from inside, or by tying it off from outside.

Frequently, it is necessary to replace the aortic valve at the same time as the mitral valve. It is usual to excise the aortic valve first so that the root can be measured, then to replace the mitral valve, and finally replace the aortic valve. If the tricuspid valve needs attention at the same operation, the right atrium can be opened with the heart beating and the aorta unclamped.

Insertion of Bjork–Shiley valve with continuous sutures

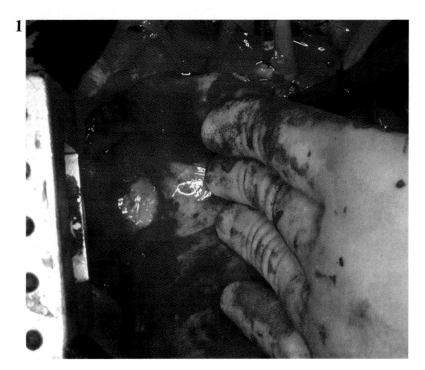

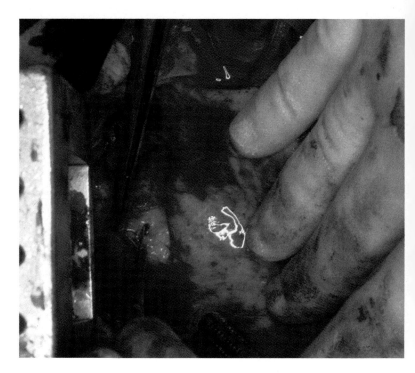

1 to 5 The approach to the mitral valve is directly through the left atrium just lateral to the interarterial groove. The initial incision is made with a knife and it is then enlarged both upwards and downwards with scissors.

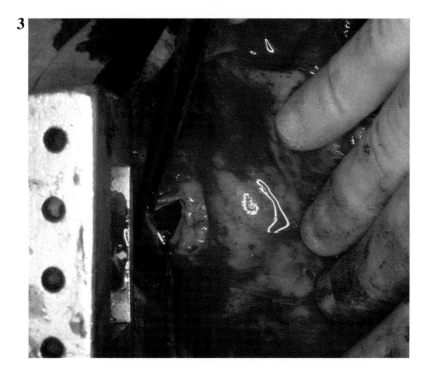

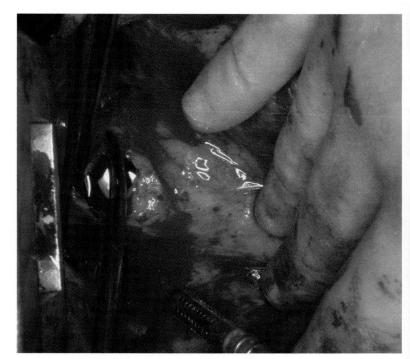

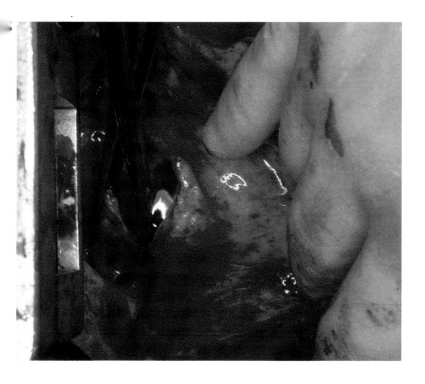

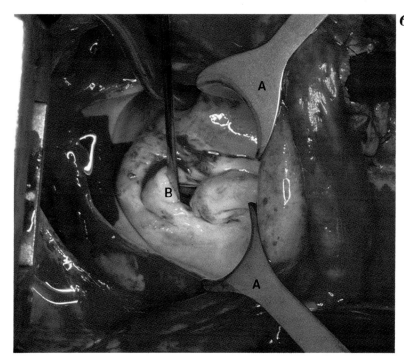

6 Retractors (**A**) pull the left atrium forwards and to the left so that the mitral valve can be seen. The posterior leaflet (**B**) is being retracted, and this pulls the whole mitral valve ring into view.

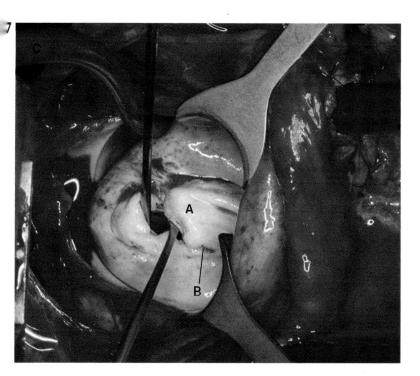

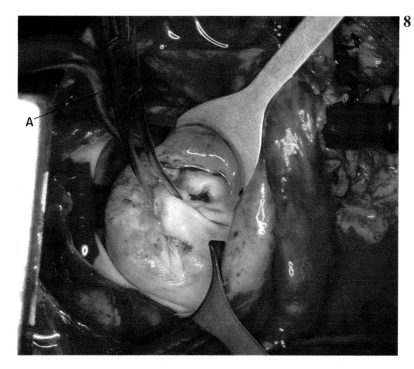

7 A second retractor is pulling on the anterior leaflet (**A**) which is rather prolapsing, and some fusion of the medial commissure is also seen (**B**). A sucking vent (**C**) returns blood to the cardiopulmonary bypass machine so as to improve the view of the valve which is often much worse than this.

8 Once the decision has been made to remove the valve rather than to repair it, the anterior leaflet is held securely with Volsellum forceps (**A**).

9

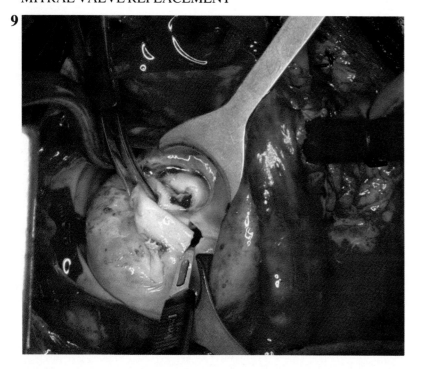

9 to 12   The anterior leaflet is first incised with a knife about 3 mm from the valve ring and the excision of the valve is then continued with scissors.

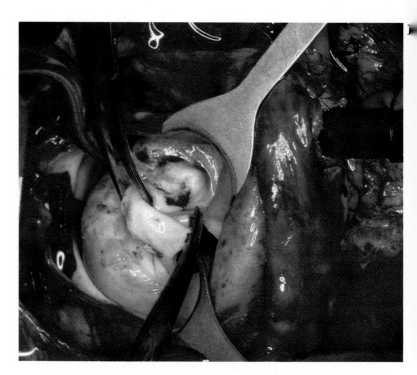

11

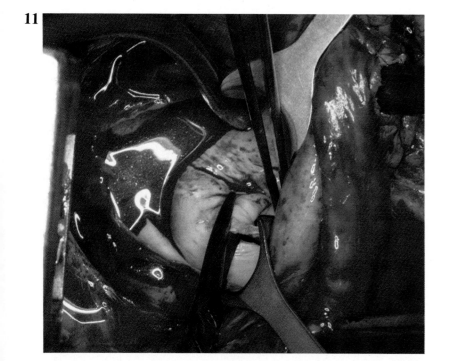

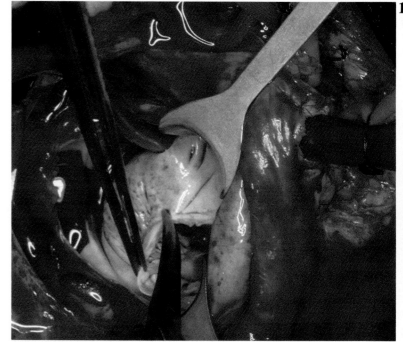

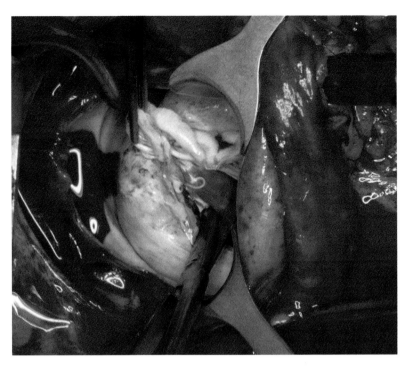

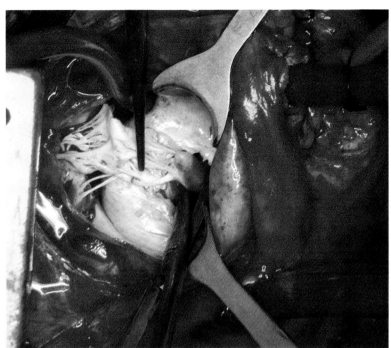

13 and 14 The papillary muscles are transected with scissors, but care must be taken not to damage the posterior wall of the left ventricle in so doing.

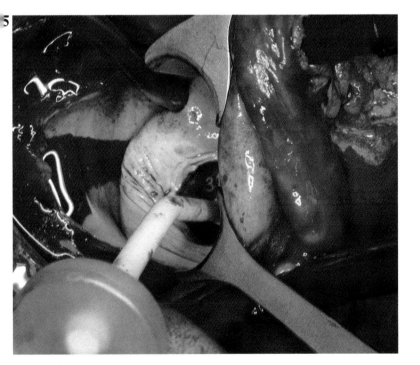

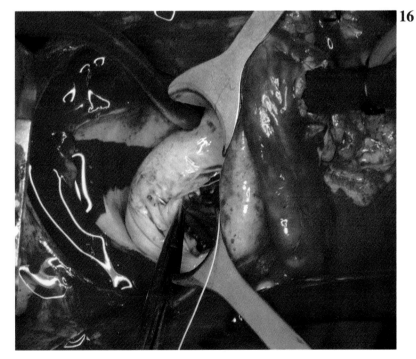

15 The size of the mitral valve ring is then measured to see what size valve should be inserted. In this case, the valve ring takes a 31 mm obturator.

16 Because this patient has a large atrium and the valve ring is well seen, it has been decided to insert a Bjork–Shiley valve with continuous sutures. The first suture is placed through the valve ring posteriorly.

17

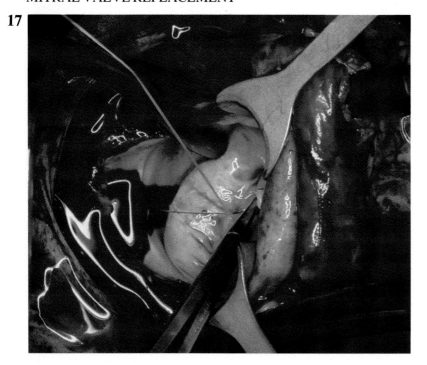

17 A second suture is placed through the valve ring anteriorly at 180° to the first suture.

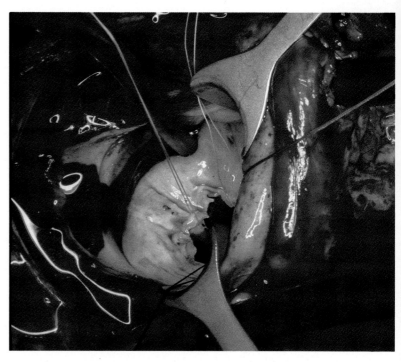

18 Two more sutures are placed through the valve ring between the first two sutures, so that the four sutures are at 90° to each other.

19

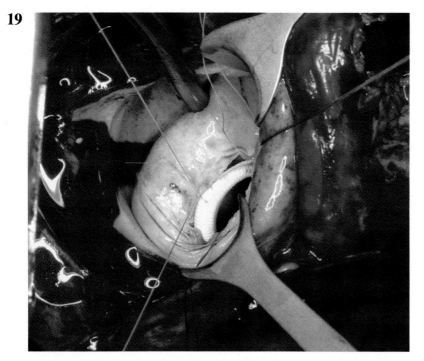

19 The posterior suture is placed through the sewing ring of the valve and the suture tied down so as to leave equal lengths of the double-ended suture. Although all four sutures can be placed through the valve at this time, it makes suturing more difficult and therefore puts more of a strain on the tissue of the valve ring.

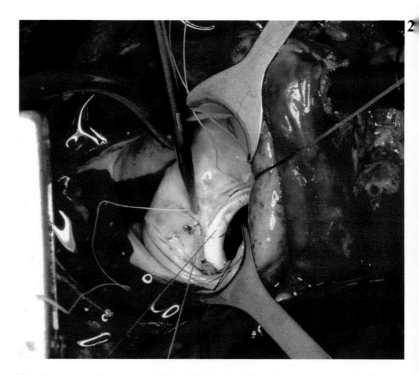

20 One suture is then carried in a clockwise direction taking a good bite of valve ring. However, the suture should not be too deep or it may be possible to damage the circumflex coronary artery.

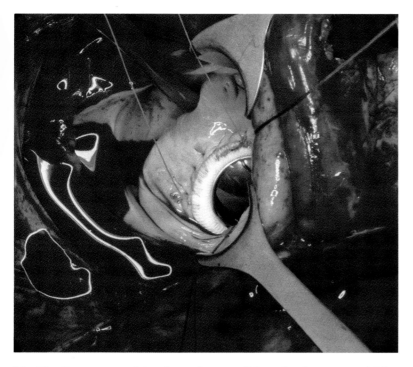

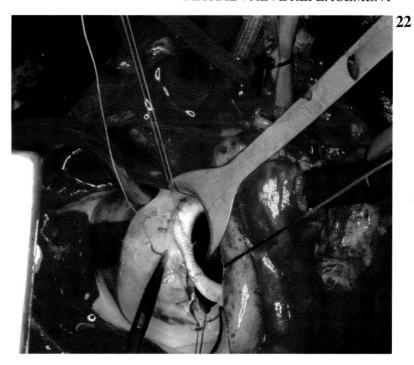

21 The first quarter of the circumference of the valve is now sutured in position.

22 to 24 The remaining quadrants of the valve are then sutured as shown.

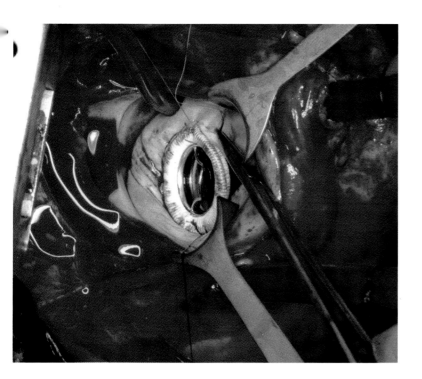

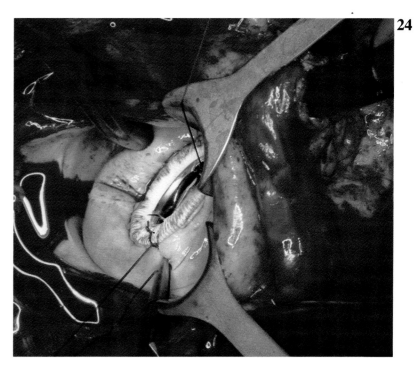

25

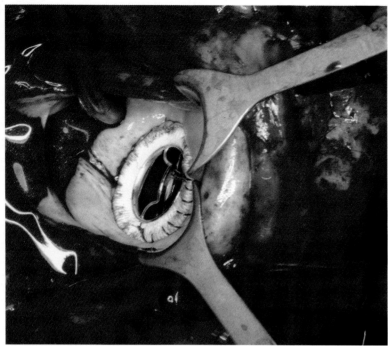

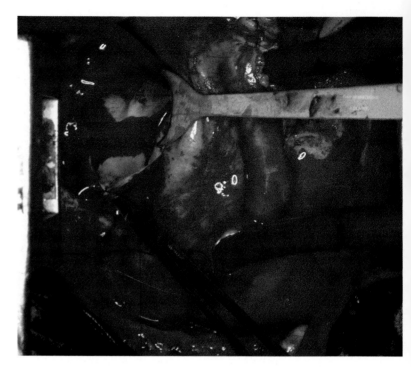

25 The valve is now completely sutured into position and it can be seen that the large orifice of the valve points backwards. This is the most commonly used position, though not essential. It is also possible to suture the valve in with a single suture, but using four sutures is probably safer, as if one quadrant pulls out, although a peripheral leak will develop, the patient should survive and present for further repair. However, if only one suture is used, a peripheral leak may be fatal.

26 to 29 Now the left atrium is closed, using continuous 3/0 Prolene. One suture is started from below and one from above; as they meet in the middle, the atrium is allowed to fill with blood to exclude air.

27

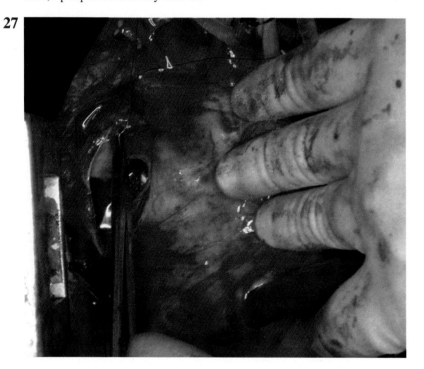

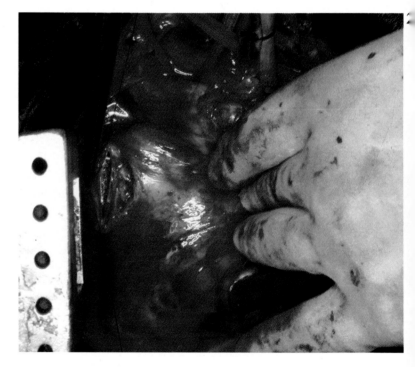

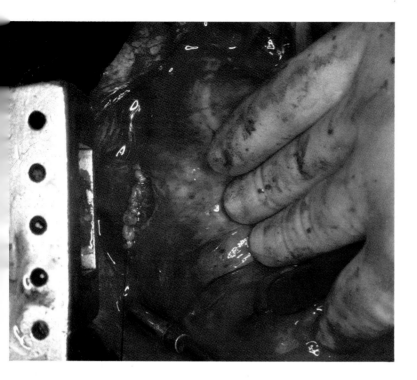

However, air will be trapped in the left ventricle and therefore, before releasing the aortic clamp, it is usual to put a needle in the left ventricular apex to vent the air. Once the aortic clamp has been released, air is further vented from the ascending aorta, by sucking with one of the open suckers on the tube used to infuse the cardioplegic solution.

Insertion of Bjork–Shiley valve with interrupted sutures

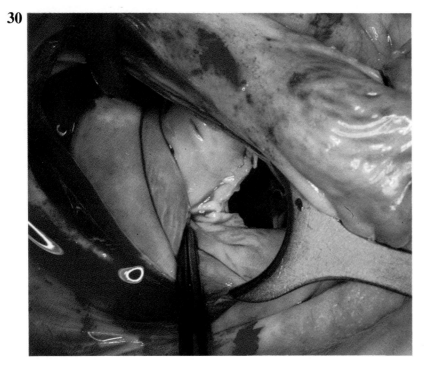

30 If the view of the valve is poor, it may be preferable to insert the valve with interrupted sutures. In this case, only the posterior part of the valve ring can be seen once the valve is excised.

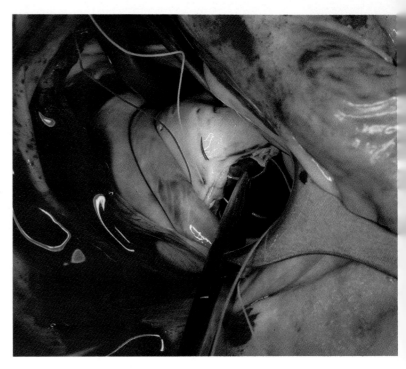

31 Starting posteriorly, a series of interrupted sutures are placed first through the sewing ring of the Bjork–Shiley valve and then through the patient's mitral valve ring. The sutures are placed first posteriorly and then, working clockwise, to the anterior part of the valve ring. Alternate white and green sutures make it easier to pick up the correct sutures to tie down later.

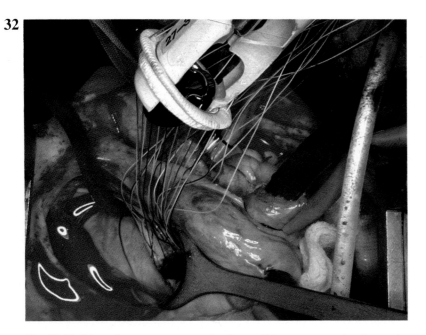

32 Half of the valve sutures are now in place, all the sutures can be clamped together and the needles cut off.

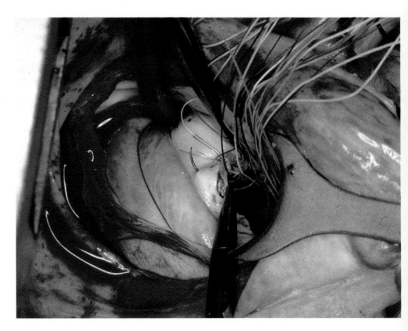

33 Starting again posteriorly, the remaining sutures are placed in an anti-clockwise direction.

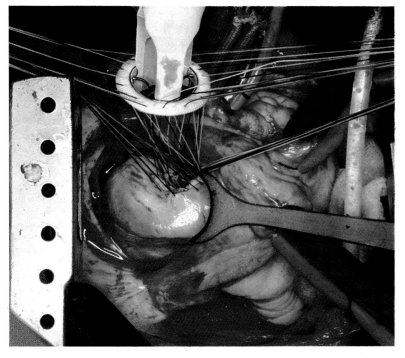
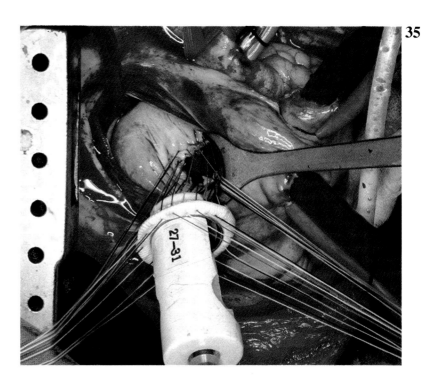

34 and 35   All the sutures are now in position.

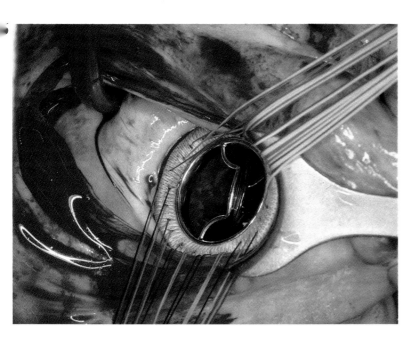
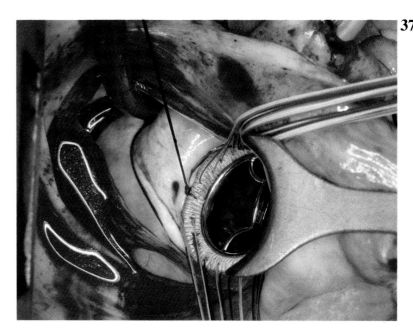

36 and 37   The valve is slid down into position, the valve holder removed and the knots tied.

38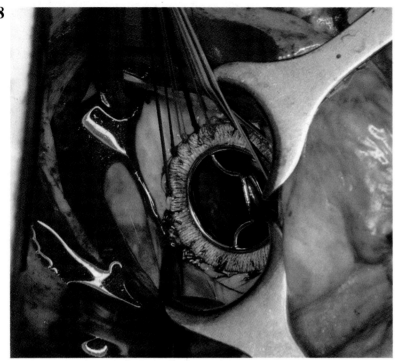

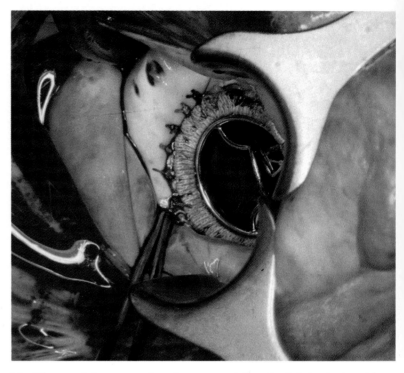

38 All the knots have been tied and half of the sutures cut.

39 The remaining sutures have been cut and the valve is in its final position ready for closure of the atrium.

Insertion of heterograft valve with continuous sutures

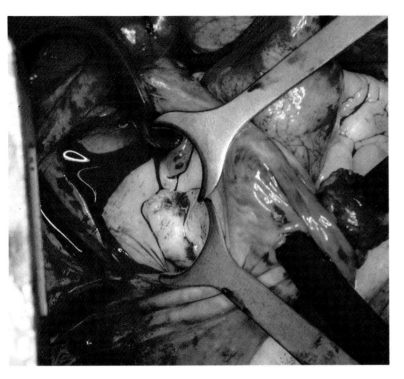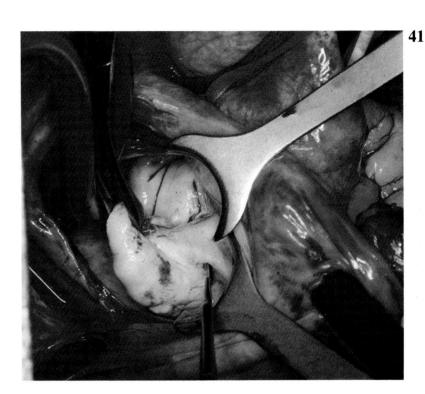

40 and 41 The anterior leaflet of the mitral valve, which is grossly prolapsing, is excised.

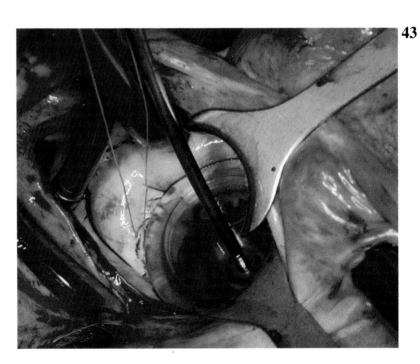

42 While the ring is pulled into view with the remnant of the posterior leaflet, a suture is placed in the posterior part of the valve ring to help retract it.

43 The valve ring is sized and the appropriate pig valve removed from its jar and washed as directed, to remove any traces of glutaraldehyde.

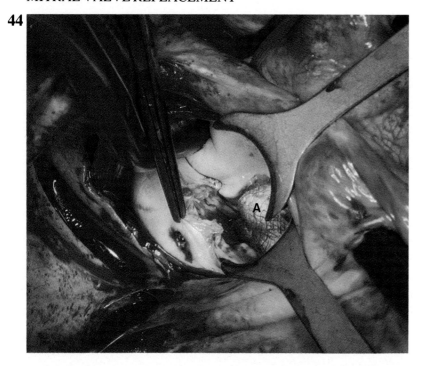

44   In this particular case, there is some calcium in the posterior part of the valve ring which needs to be removed. A swab (**A**) has been temporarily placed in the left ventricle to catch any little pieces of the friable calcium.

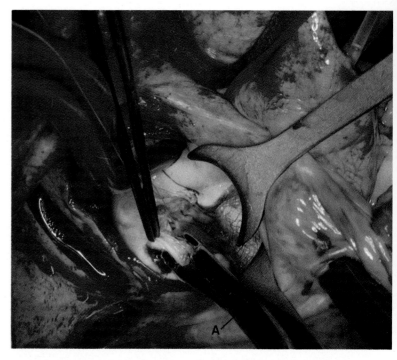

45   The calcium is being removed with a pair of Caldwell–Luc forceps (**A**).

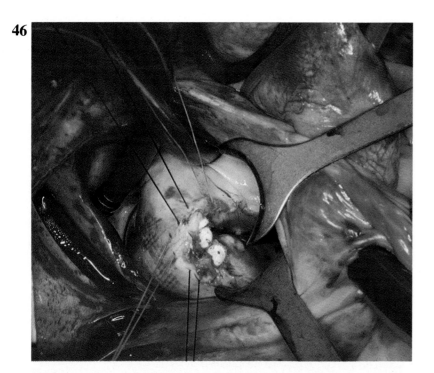

46   In this case, it was felt that removing the calcium had slightly weakened the valve ring in that region and therefore three mattress sutures on pledgets of Teflon felt were inserted to support the weakened area.

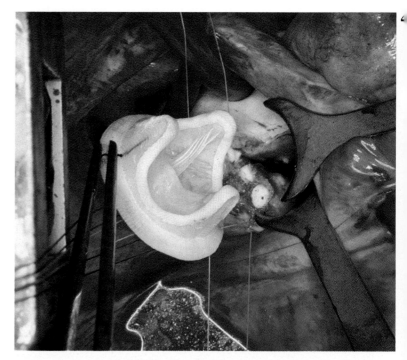

47   These sutures are then placed through the sewing ring of a pig valve which is then inverted into the left ventricle.

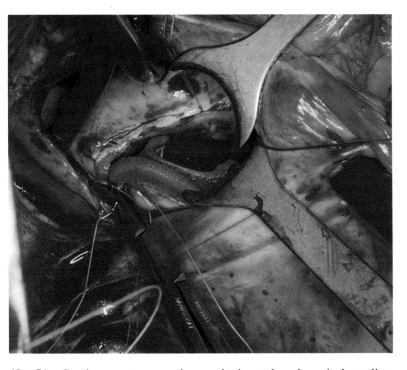

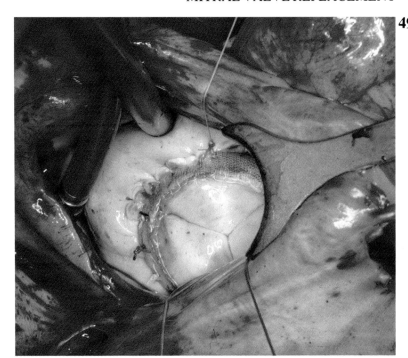

48 to 51   Continuous sutures are then used to insert the valve as in the earlier part of the chapter.

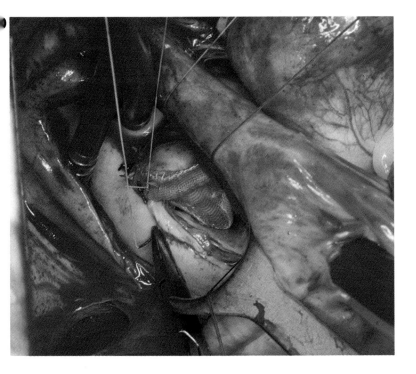

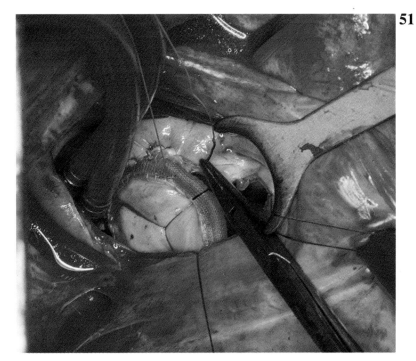

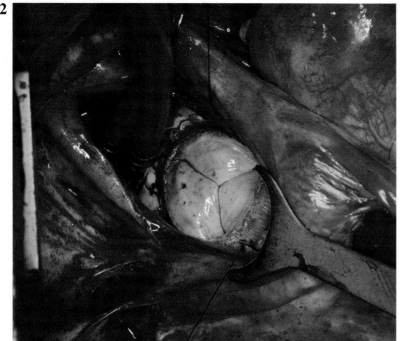

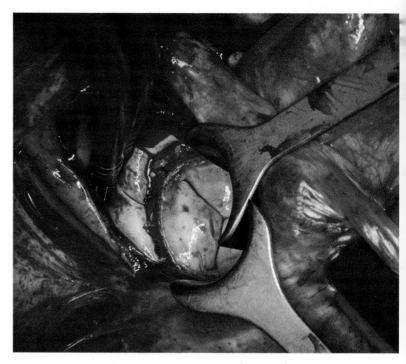

52 The final quadrant is about to be sutured into position.

53 The final position of the valve is seen before closure of the atrium.

7: Tricuspid annuloplasty

Regurgitation of the tricuspid valve may be caused by back pressure due to mitral valve disease. This functional regurgitation, as it is called, is due to enlargement of the right ventricle and stretching of the valve ring and the tricuspid valve apparatus. The cusps themselves are not diseased, and therefore if the valve ring is constricted, the valve can become competent again. This is not the case with organic tricuspid regurgitation, when the valve cusps are diseased and may need replacing rather than repair.

If the valve ring is to be narrowed, it must be remembered that the septal portion of the tricuspid valve ring is immobile, and furthermore contains the conducting mechanism of the heart. Several different types of tricuspid annuloplasty have been used. The Carpentier ring[1] is well tried and involves the insertion of a cloth-covered metal ring which is carefully sized so that the septal portion of the tricuspid valve ring is not altered, but the rest of the ring is pulled in when the ring is inserted. The principle is the same as for the insertion of a ring into the mitral position (see Chapter 5).

A cheaper and easier technique is that introduced by De Vega[2] which results in the same pulling in of the parietal portion of the tricuspid annulus, but this is achieved with one Prolene suture. The stitch is inserted under direct vision, but tied down after bypass has been discontinued with the surgeon's finger in the atrium. This allows the ring to be narrowed until no more regurgitation can be felt.[3]

Nearly always, tricuspid annuloplasty is performed at the same time as mitral and/or aortic valve surgery.

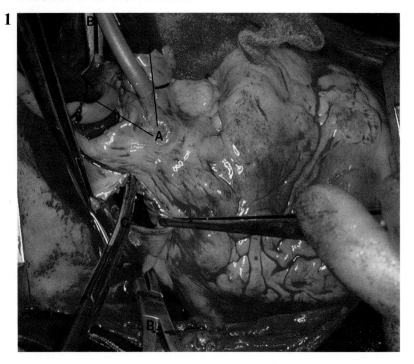

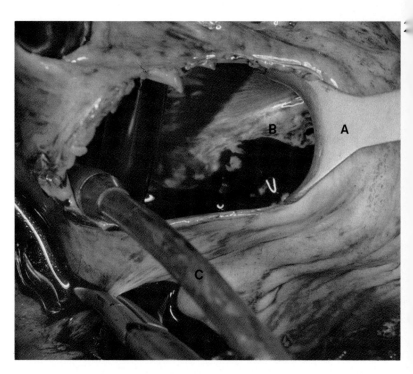

1 Venous cannulae (**A**) are inserted into the venae cavae and snugged with Cooley clamps (**B**) and the right atrium is opened with a pair of scissors (**C**).

2 A retractor (**A**) exposes the tricuspid valve (**B**) and blood is sucked from the right atrium back to the heart-lung machine with one of the open suckers (**C**). In this case, the annuloplasty is being performed with the heart beating and therefore a lot of blood will be returning to the right atrium via the coronary sinus.

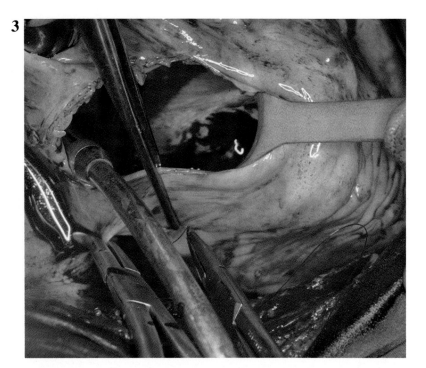

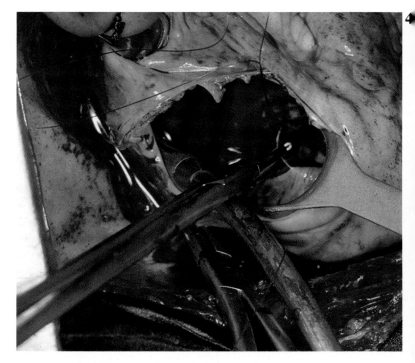

3 A 3/0 Prolene suture is placed from outside the inferior wall of the right atrium into the interior of the right atrium at the inferior border of the valve ring at the junction of the septal and inferior leaflets of the tricuspid valve. Care must be taken not to damage the right coronary artery.

4 The suture is then continued in an anti-clockwise direction in and out of the valve ring.

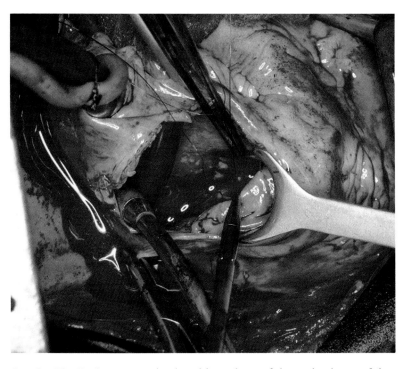

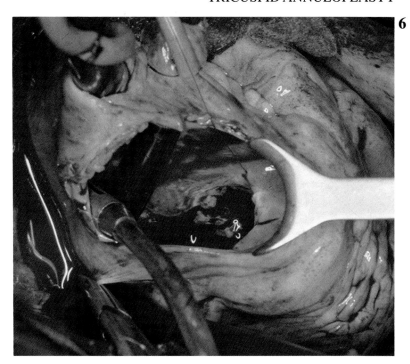

5 to 7 The Prolene suture is placed in and out of the parietal part of the tricuspid valve ring anteriorly as far as the junction of the anterior and septal leaflets.

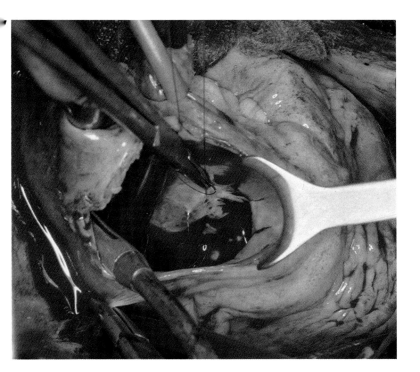

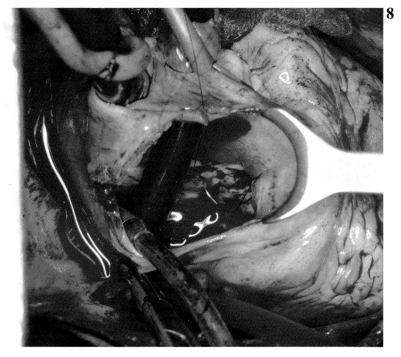

8 The suture is then reversed and the needle can be seen here starting on the return journey in a clockwise direction around the same part of the tricuspid valve ring.

9

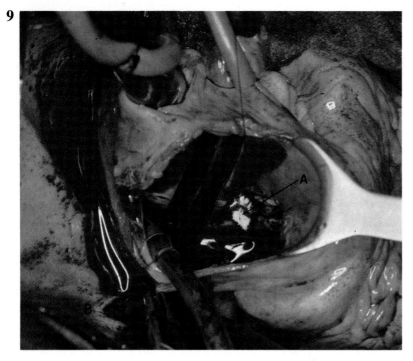

9 To prevent the suture from cutting through, it is passed through a small piece of Teflon felt (**A**). It is a wise precaution to fix this felt to the tricuspid valve ring with a suture (**B**), so that if the Prolene suture were to break, the felt would not be carried into the pulmonary artery.

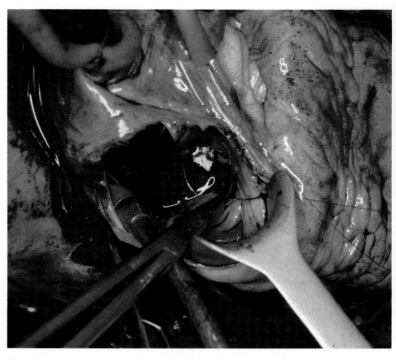

10 The return journey of the suture anteriorly around the tricuspid valve ring has been completed and the needle brought out close to where the suture started on the valve ring.

11

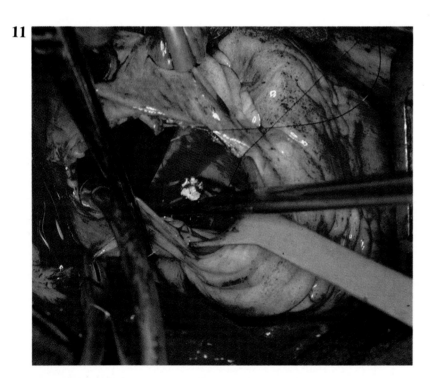

11 The needle is then passed through to the outside of the right atrium, again taking care to avoid the right coronary artery.

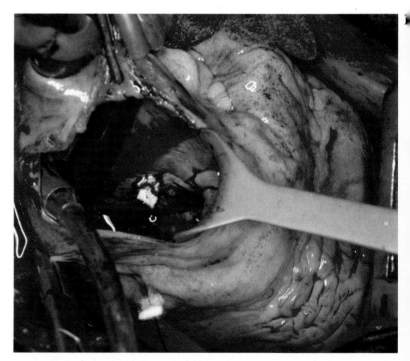

12 The two needles of the double-ended Prolene suture are passed through another piece of Teflon felt which will prevent the suture cutting through the atrial wall when the knot is tied.

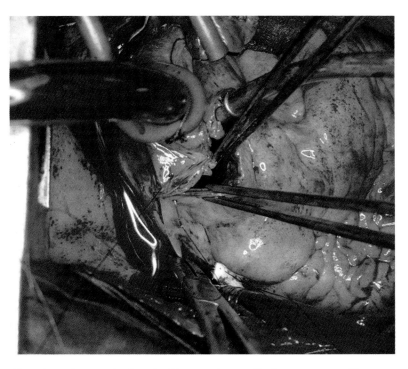

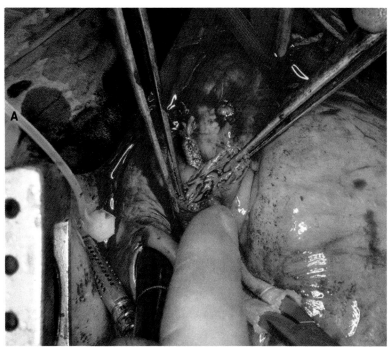

13 The atriotomy is closed with a continuous Prolene suture and bypass discontinued.

14 One venous cannula has been removed from the right atrial appendage, which is occluded with a Brock clamp. The left atrial pressure is being monitored through the pressure line (**A**).

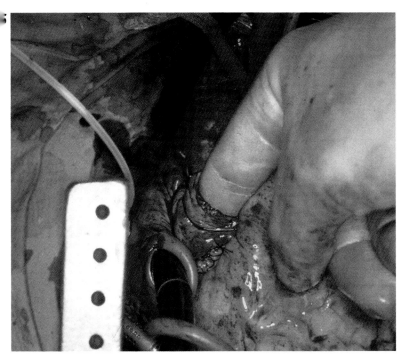

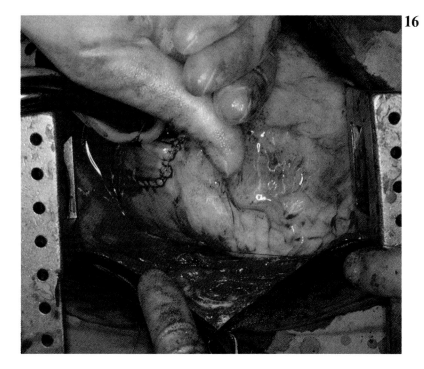

15 and 16 The finger is inserted into the right atrial appendage and while this finger assesses the tricuspid regurgitation, the assistant ties the Prolene suture down on to the Teflon felt until the tricuspid ring has been narrowed just enough to stop the regurgitation. The finger is then removed, the atrial appendage tied and the heart decannulated.

8: Tricuspid valve replacement

Where possible, the tricuspid valve should be conserved (see Chapter 7). However, when it is severely affected by the rheumatic process, satisfactory repair may be impossible. Other rarer conditions may affect the tricuspid valve necessitating replacement, such as the carcinoid syndrome, as in the patient whose tricuspid valve replacement is illustrated in this chapter.

There is still no ideal valve substitute for the tricuspid valve, but it has been shown that some prosthetic valves have an unacceptably high incidence of thrombosis in the tricuspid position[1] despite adequate anticoagulation and, therefore, a tissue valve, such as the pig valve shown in this chapter, is preferable.

It is unusual to have to replace only the tricuspid valve, and frequently the mitral, and occasionally the aortic, valve also need attention.

The approach is through a midline sternotomy (see Chapter 2) and cardiopulmonary bypass is used. Two separate caval cannulae are needed with caval snugging, but it is unnecessary to clamp the aorta, and the valve replacement can be performed as shown in this chapter, with the heart beating.

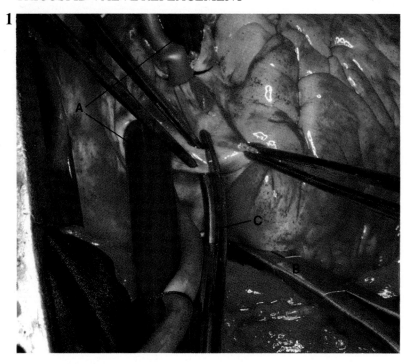

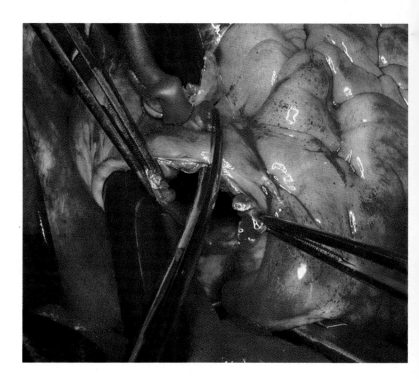

1 and 2 Venous cannulae (**A**) are inserted into the venae cavae and snugged with Cooley clamps (**B**). The right atrium is opened with scissors (**C**) and the incision enlarged.

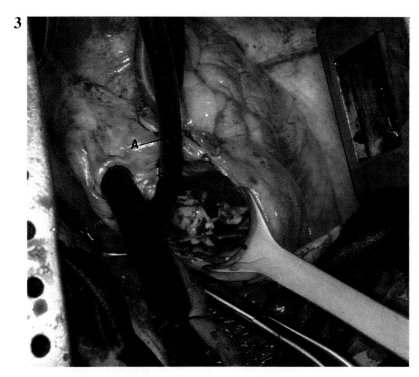

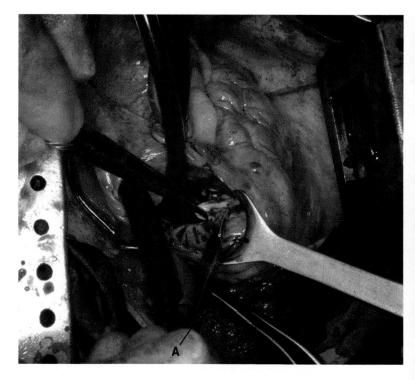

3 The abnormal tricuspid valve is revealed with retraction and a suction tube (**A**) returns blood from the coronary sinus to the heart–lung machine. The tricuspid valve in this patient has been grossly affected by the carcinoid syndrome and is quite unsuitable for repair.

4 The valve is being excised, starting anteriorly with a knife (**A**).

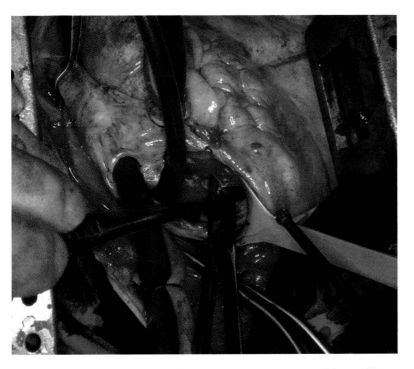

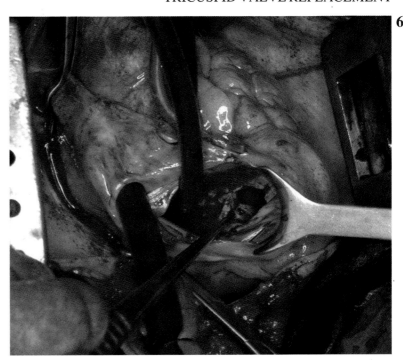

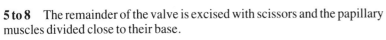

5 to 8 The remainder of the valve is excised with scissors and the papillary muscles divided close to their base.

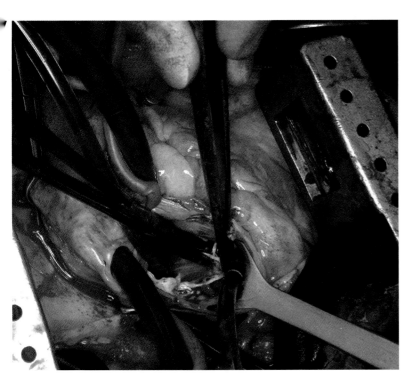

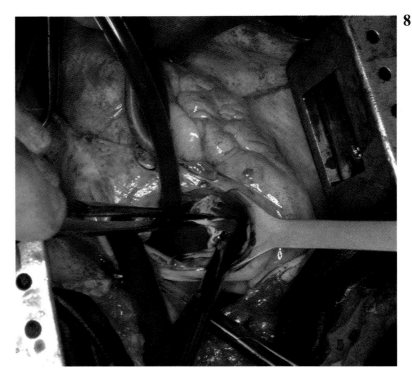

9

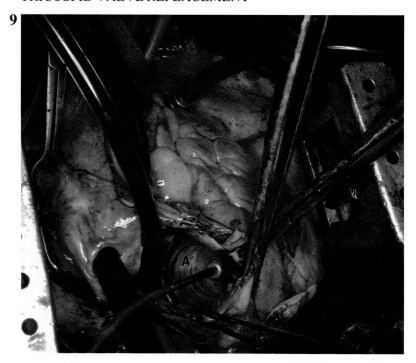

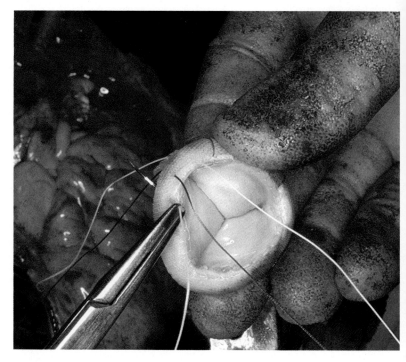

9 The size of the valve ring is measured with an obturator (**A**) to judge what size valve is needed.

10 to 12 A pig valve is inserted using interrupted sutures posteriorly on the septum, which are tied down. A suture is left long on each side and the remainder of the valve can be sutured in continuously.

11

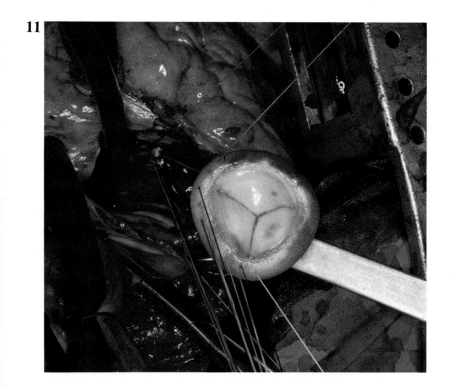

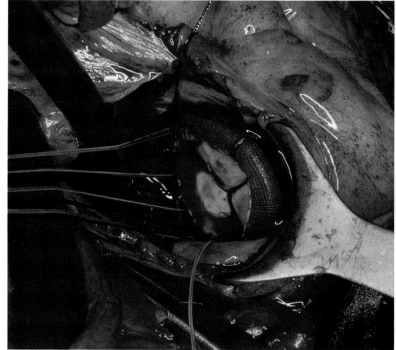

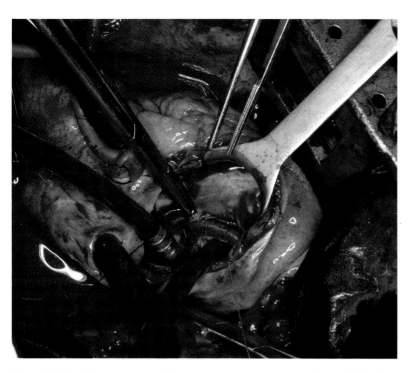

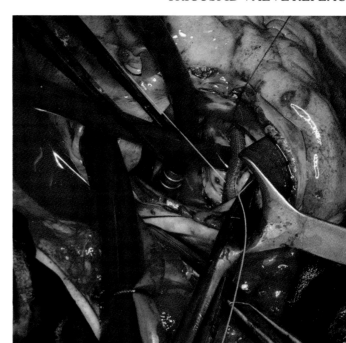

13 and 14 The two remaining sutures are run around anteriorly to complete the insertion.

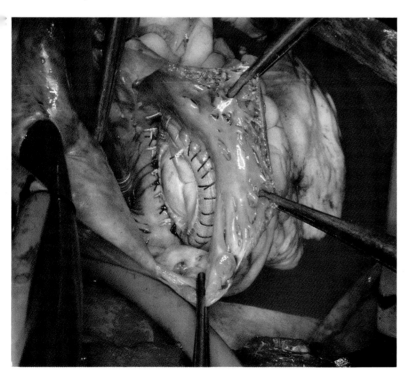

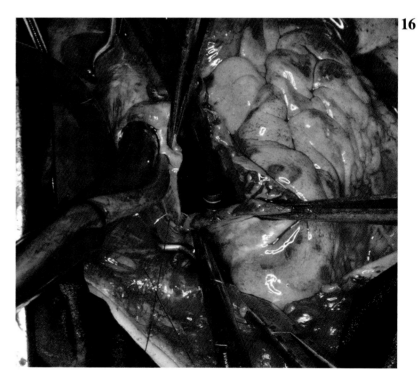

15 The final appearance of the valve in position is shown. This is, in fact, a different patient.

16 Finally, with the valve in position, the right atrium is closed, the venae cavae unsnugged and cardiopulmonary bypass discontinued.

9: Coronary artery bypass grafting

Direct revascularisation of the coronary arteries was introduced in the late 1960s[1] and has become the commonest procedure in cardiac surgery. Reversed autogenous long saphenous vein is the most commonly used graft material, and is placed from the aorta as a bypass to the appropriate coronary artery or arteries beyond the narrowing. Internal mammary artery may also be used either as a free graft or still attached proximally.

It is essential to the planning of coronary artery bypass grafts to know the exact extent of disease, and the surgeon must have good quality coronary angiograms to guide him. Clearly, the distal end of the graft must be anastomosed to a suitable place on the coronary artery beyond the narrowing, and the proximal end of the graft is anastomosed to the ascending aorta.

The operation is performed through a median sternotomy and, although the heart itself is not opened, it is usual to use cardiopulmonary bypass in order to secure a still, dry heart for the performance of the delicate distal anastomoses.

The coronary artery anatomy can be quite variable but a typical pattern is shown in diagram **A**. A hypothetical but common distribution of disease is shown in diagram **B**, together with the siting of the vein bypass grafts.

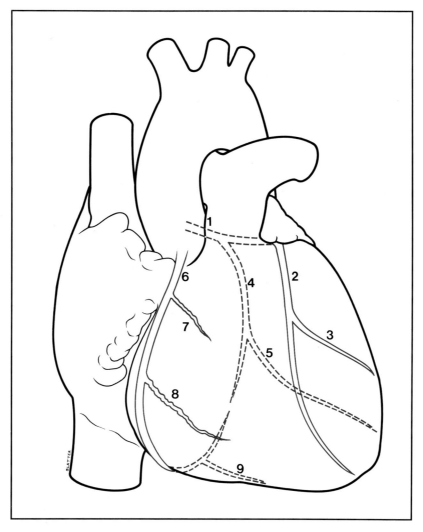

Diagram A
1. Left main.
2. Left anterior descending (LAD).
3. Diagonal.
4. Circumflex.
5. Obtuse marginal.
6. Right.
7. Right ventricular branch.
8. Acute marginal branch.
9. Posterior interventricular.

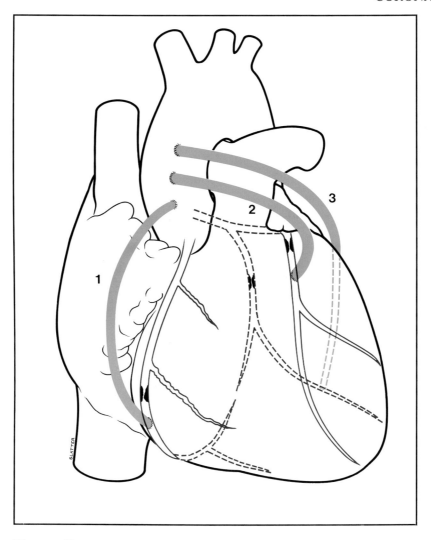

Diagram B
1. Graft to right coronary artery.
2. Graft to left anterior descending coronary artery.
3. Graft to obtuse marginal branch of circumflex coronary artery.

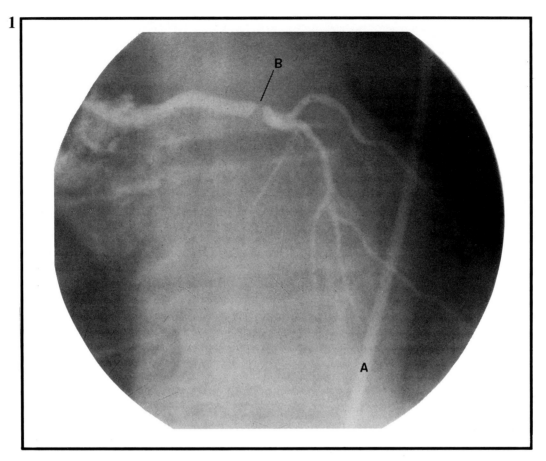

1 This is a left coronary angiogram which has been performed by passing a catheter (**A**) into the femoral artery, up the aorta and round into the ascending aorta, from where the appropriate coronary artery is entered. An injection of dye has shown the left main coronary artery to have a virtual occlusion (**B**) and further ragged disease in the left coronary artery.

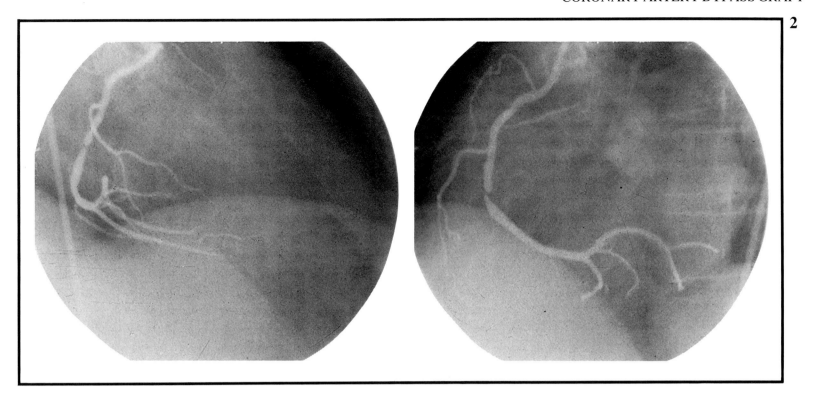

2   Two views of the right coronary artery are seen. On the left, the view has been taken from the right side of the patient (right anterior oblique) and the right hand picture has been taken in the left anterior oblique position. They show a 90% stenosis in the mid-portion of the artery with a good distal vessel.

Removal of long saphenous vein

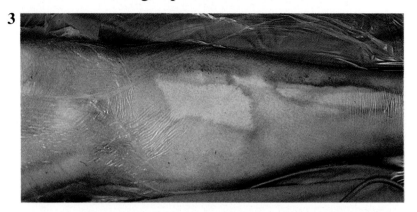 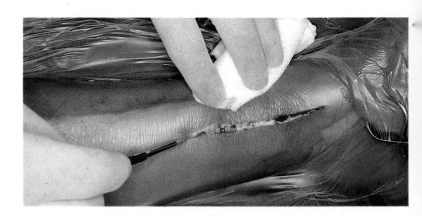

3 and 4 The leg is suitably prepared at the same time as the chest and it is customary for an assistant to remove the vein at the same time as the surgeon opens the chest. In this case, the vein is being removed below the knee.

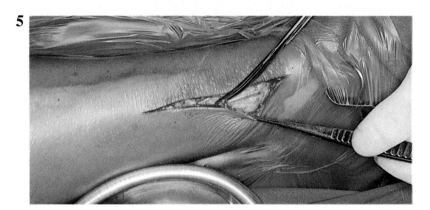 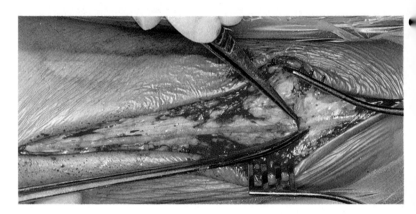

5 to 8 The required length of vein is dissected free.

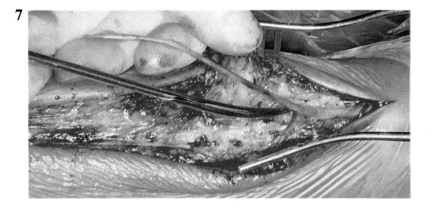 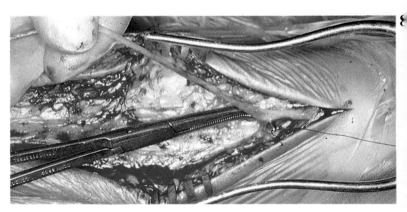

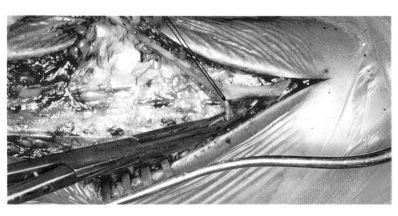

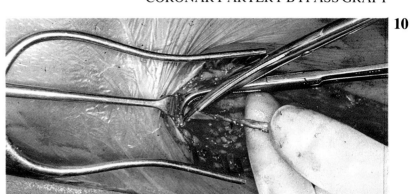

9 and 10 All branches must be tied or clipped, and when the appropriate length has been freed, the vein is clamped and cut free, taking care to remember which end is which. The cut end of vein remaining in the patient is tied off.

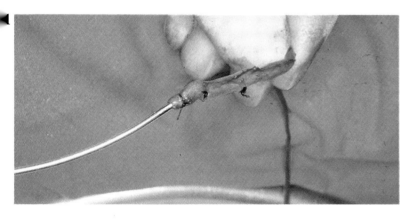

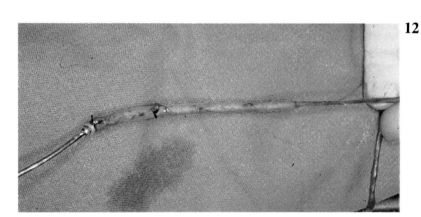

11 and 12 A cannula is then tied into the distal end of the vein and the vein is gently distended. Excessive pressure may damage the intima of the vein. The vein is then ready for use.

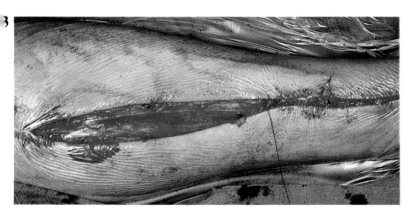

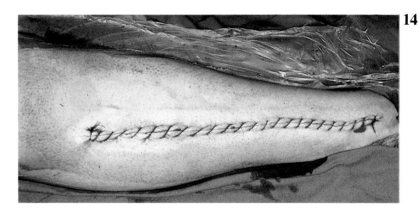

13 and 14 The leg wound is then closed with a subcutaneous continuous catgut suture and the skin with continuous monofilament nylon. Commonly, the leg wound is packed with a wet swab during the bypass procedure and closed when the chest is being closed.

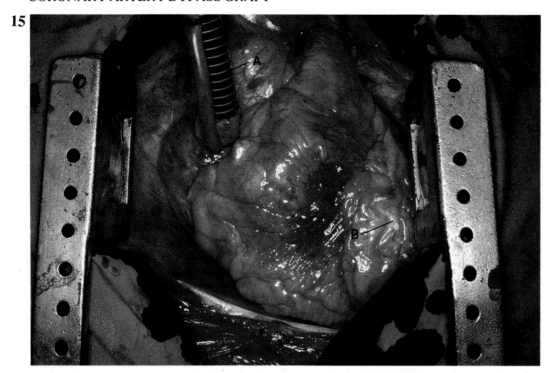

15 While the assistant is removing the vein from the leg, the surgeon opens the chest and prepares for institution of cardiopulmonary bypass (see Chapter 2). The single venous cannula can be seen (**A**), and the tortuous left anterior descending (LAD) coronary artery is clearly seen (**B**).

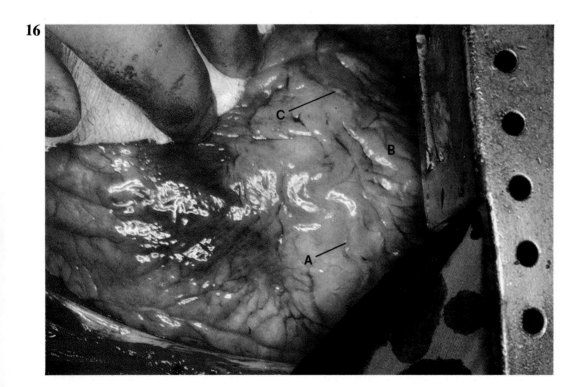

16 Retraction of the heart gives a better exposure of the LAD coronary artery (**A**) and its diagonal branch (**B**). Atheroma (**C**) can be seen proximally in the diagonal vessel.

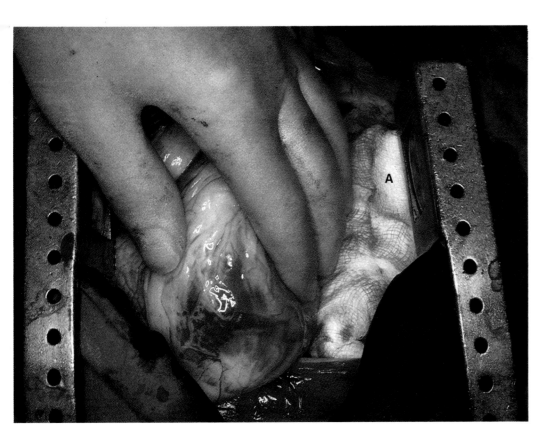

17 The heart must be still for the intricate distal anastomosis. Therefore cardiopulmonary bypass is commenced, the aorta cross-clamped and cardioplegic solution infused into the ascending aorta (see Chapter 1). The exposure is made easier by placing a large swab (**A**) behind the heart.

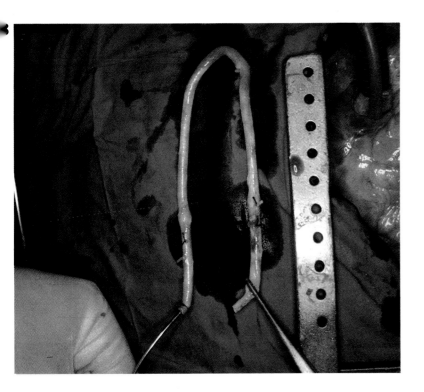

18 The long saphenous vein which has been dissected out by the assistant is checked for any leaks.

Grafting to the left anterior descending coronary artery

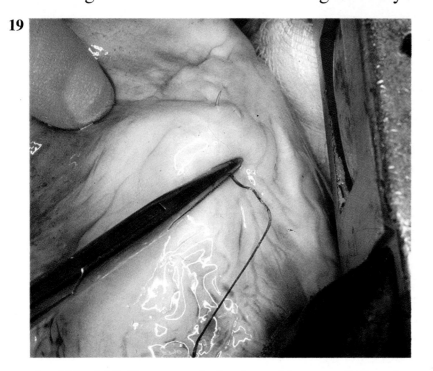

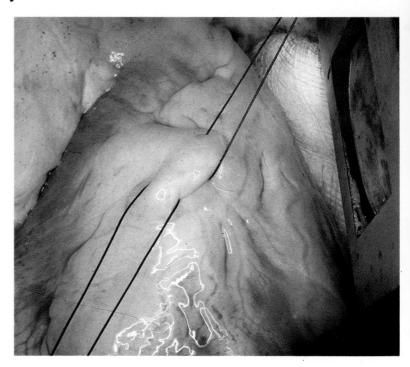

19 and 20   A 2/0 silk stay suture is placed around the artery, which can be quite difficult to see once the cardioplegia has washed out the blood.

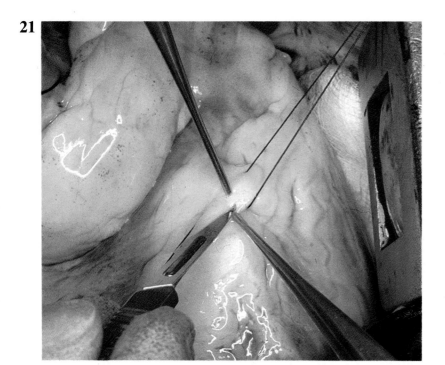

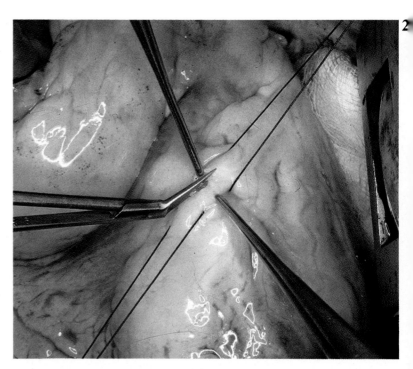

21   The initial incision in the artery is made with a sharp knife, taking care not to damage the back wall of the artery.

22   The incision is then enlarged with fine scissors.

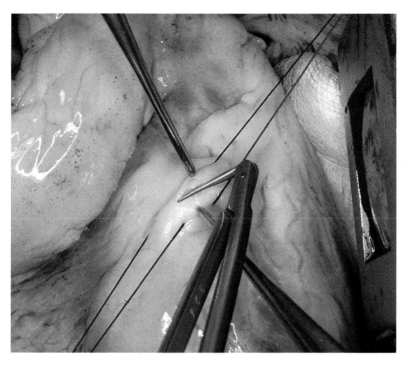

23 Reversed scissors are helpful to enlarge the incision in the other direction.

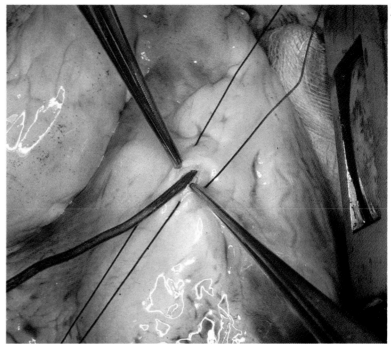

24 Graduated probes can be passed into the artery to measure the internal diameter, which in this case is 2 mm. The probes are also helpful in detecting narrowings in the vessel and distal patency.

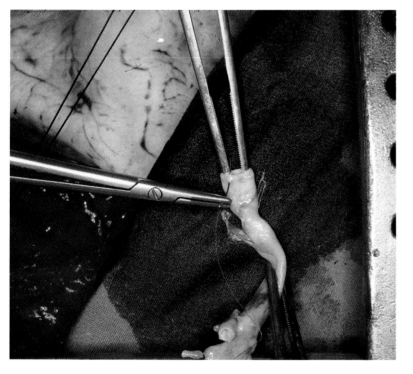

25 The anastomosis is then begun. It is helpful to place some sutures in the vein and artery before sliding the vein down on to the artery. This allows the surgeon to see the end of the arteriotomy clearly for the careful placement of the most important end sutures. Here the 7/0 Prolene stitch is first placed into the vein which is held on the side towel.

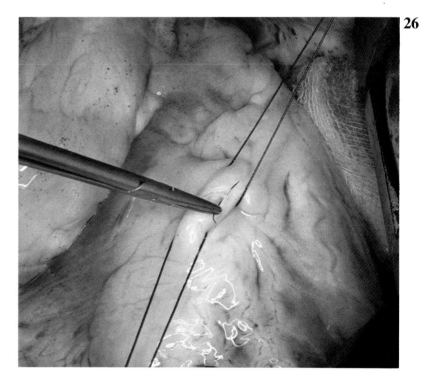

26 The next suture is placed just medial to the proximal end of the arteriotomy.

27

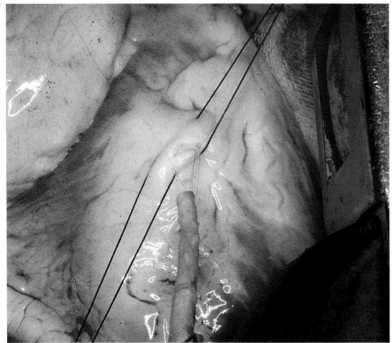

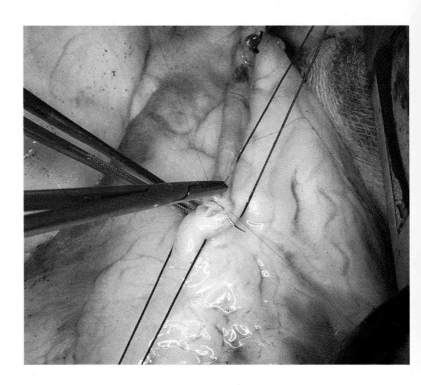

27 Two further bites of this continuous suture are inserted before sliding the vein down into position.

29

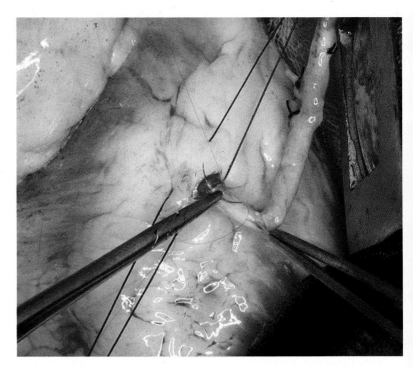

28 to 30 The remainder of the anastomosis is completed with the lateral end of the 7/0 Prolene suture. It is helpful to have pulled this through more than the other end when sliding down the vein as it makes the following easier. Simultaneous bites through the vein and artery may be taken except at

the distal end, where it is usually advisable to insert the needle first through the vein and pull it through, and then insert it into the artery. The distal end of the arteriotomy is the most likely to be narrowed in the anastomosis and therefore very small bites must be taken at this point.

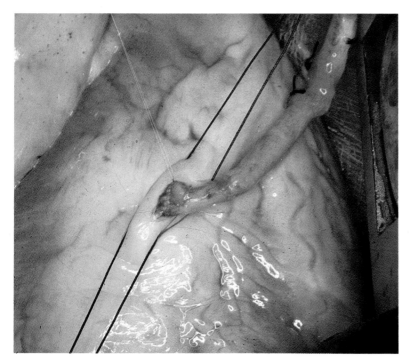

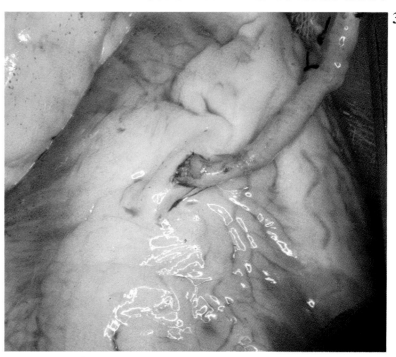

31 and 32   Once the continuous suture has been inserted, the knot is tied and the suture is cut. In using Prolene, which is designed to pull through very easily, care must be taken not to tie the knot too tight and thus narrow the anastomosis by purse-stringing it.

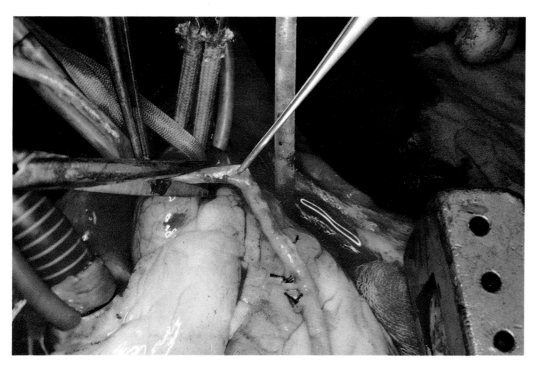

33   The vein is then gently pulled up towards the aorta and cut at what is judged to be the correct point, thus leaving exactly enough vein so that the vein will be neither too taut nor redundant.

Grafting to the right coronary artery

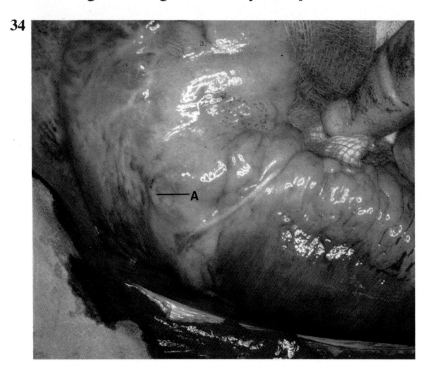

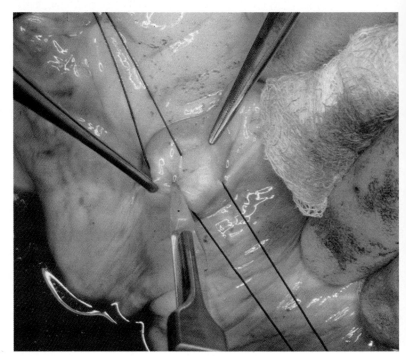

34 The heart is held forwards with a swab and the right coronary artery, which is usually buried in fat, can just be seen (**A**).

35 and 36 Again, the 2/0 silk sutures are placed around the artery and an incision is made in it.

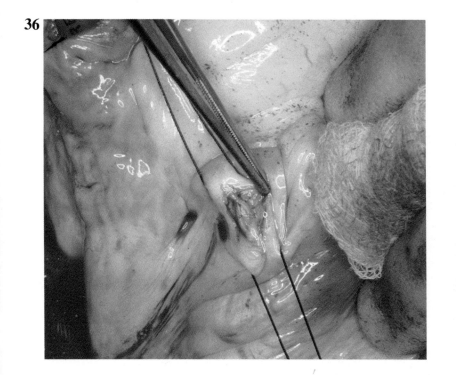

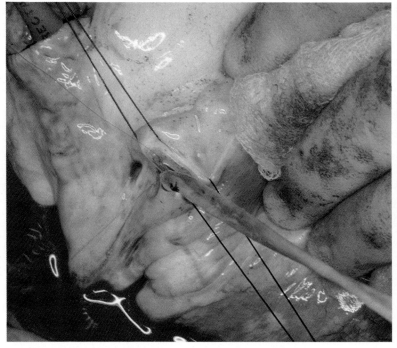

37 to 40 Again using 7/0 Prolene, the distal anastomosis of the vein to the artery is made.

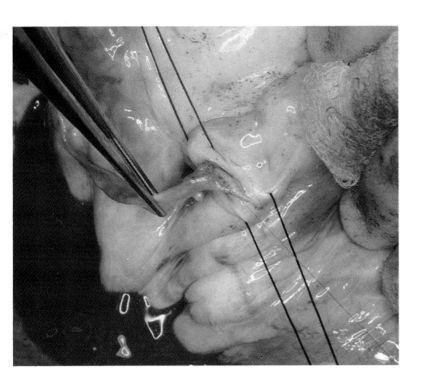

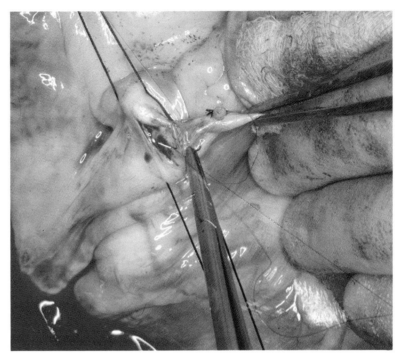

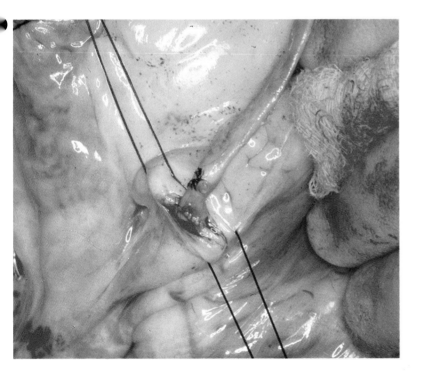

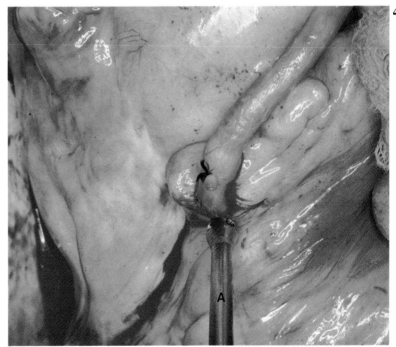

41 Having finished the distal anastomoses (in this case LAD and right coronary arteries), the aortic clamp is released and the graft fills with back bleeding. A sucker (**A**) is just removing some blood and the anastomoses are checked for leaks.

42

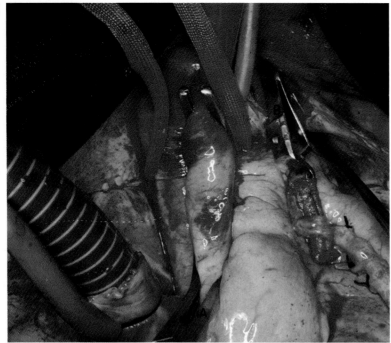

42 The proximal anastomoses are then performed with the heart normally perfused and beating. A side-clamp (**A**) is applied to the ascending aorta. The vein graft to the LAD coronary artery is seen, the back bleeding having been stopped by clamping it with a bull-dog clamp (**B**).

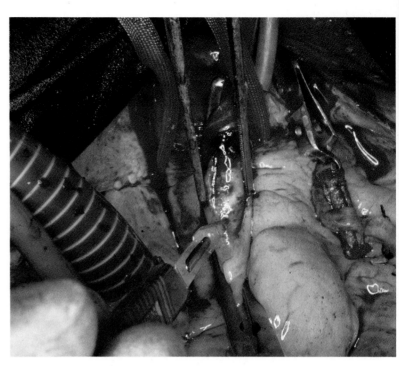

43 The adventitia of the selected part of the ascending aorta is removed and a hole made with a knife where each proximal anastomosis is to be.

44

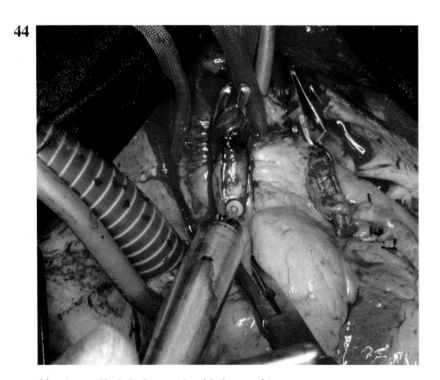

44 A round hole is then made with the punch.

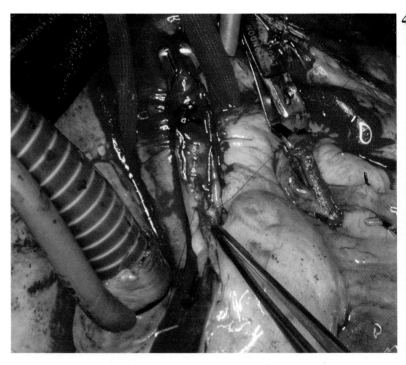

45 to 48 The proximal end of vein graft to the right coronary artery is then performed with 5/0 Prolene.

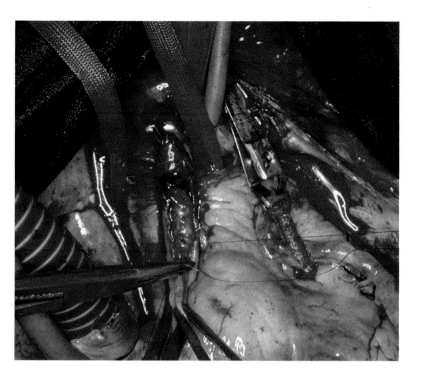
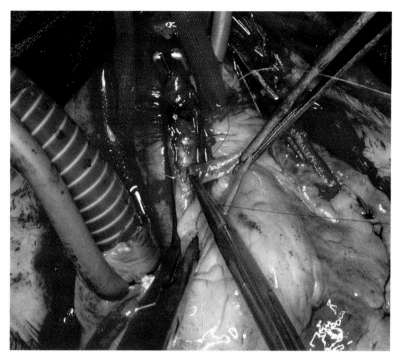

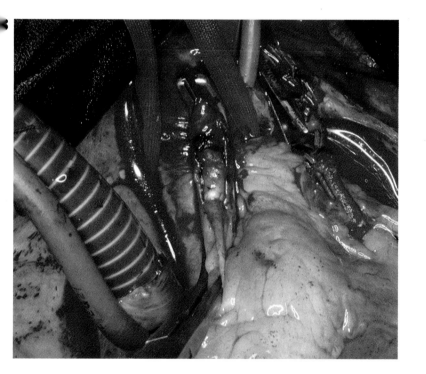
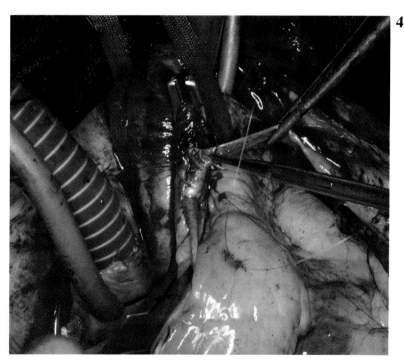

49 The proximal anastomosis of the graft to the LAD coronary artery is performed above the right coronary artery graft, again using 5/0 Prolene.

50

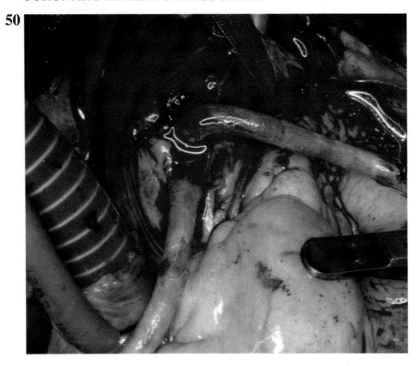

50 The aortic side-clamp is then released and the grafts promptly fill.

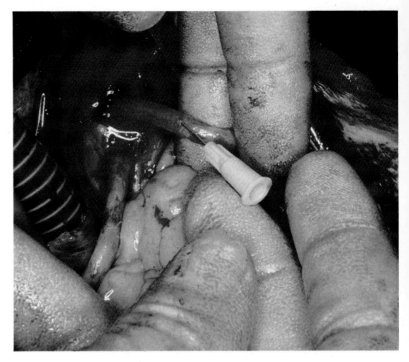

51 However, air may be trapped in the proximal part of the vein graft and this is removed with a fine bore needle before releasing the bull-dog clamp. Cardiopulmonary bypass is now stopped and the heart takes over the circulation completely.

52

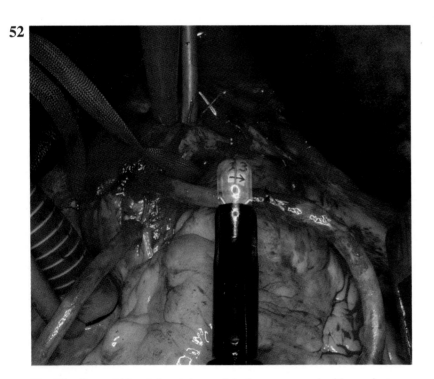

52 The flow of blood down the graft is then measured with an electro-magnetic flow probe.

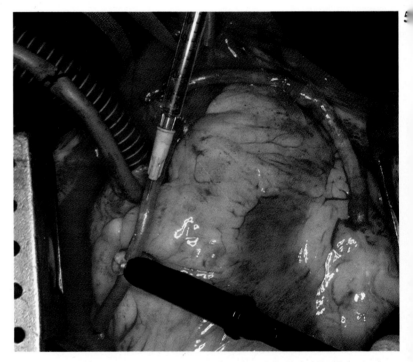

53 While the flow is still measured, papaverine can be injected down the vein to cause vasodilatation in the distal artery. If there is a good run-off and the anastomosis is not obstructing, the flow down the graft usually doubles.

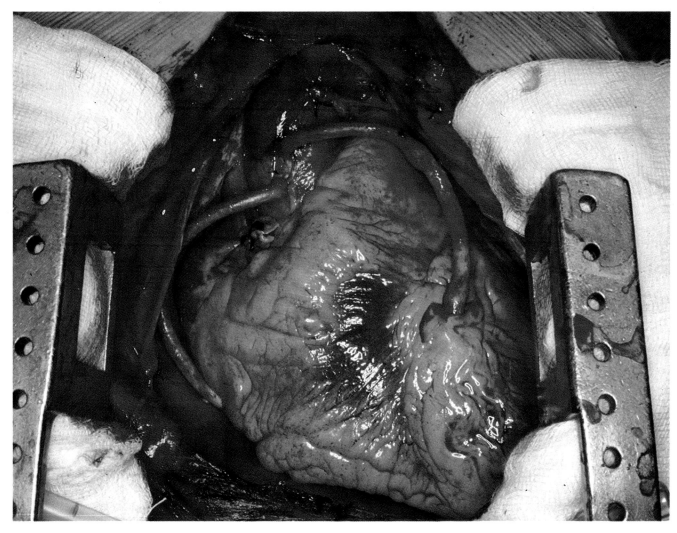

54 Just before closing the chest, the grafts to the right and LAD coronary arteries are checked to ensure that there is no leak from the anastomoses.

Grafting to obtuse marginal branch of circumflex coronary artery

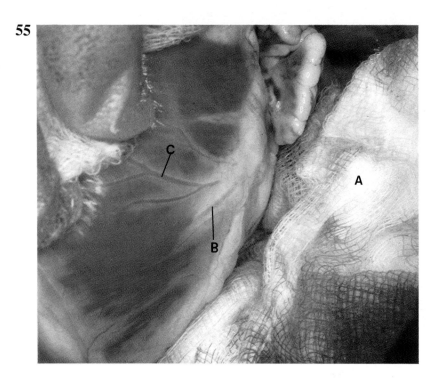

55   The main circumflex coronary artery is extremely difficult to reach as it lies in the fat in the atrioventricular groove, and usually one of its obtuse marginal branches arising distal to the stenosis is selected for grafting. Even so, the exposure is still difficult and is helped by placing a swab behind the heart (**A**). The obtuse marginal artery (**B**) can be seen emerging from the fat of the atrioventricular groove and must not be confused with a coronary vein (**C**).

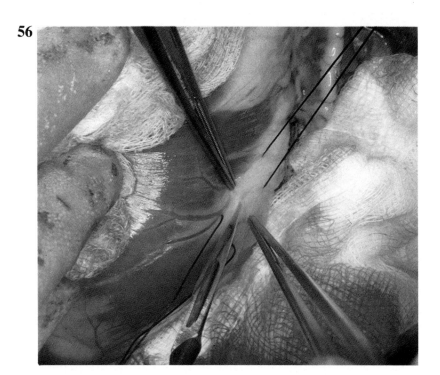

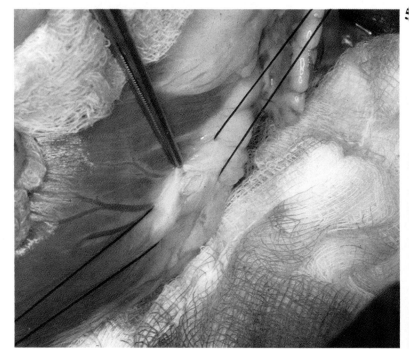

56 and 57   Stay sutures are placed around the artery which is incised as before.

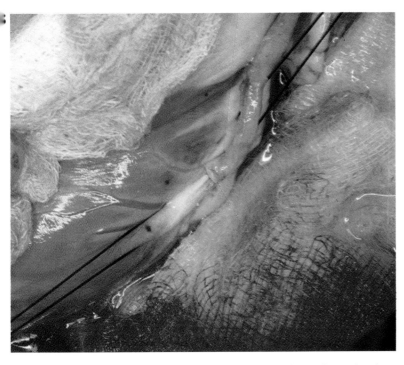

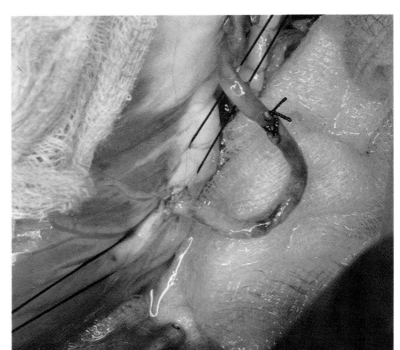

58 to 61   The distal anastomosis of the vein is again performed using continuous 7/0 Prolene.

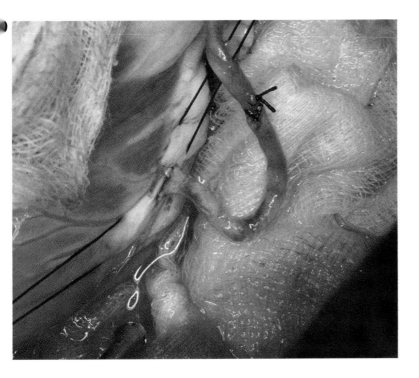

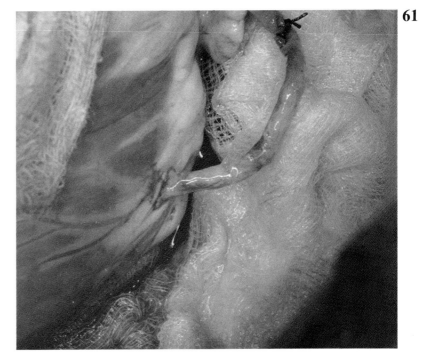

Endarterectomy of right coronary artery

62

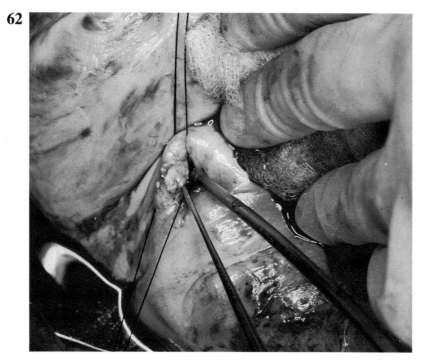

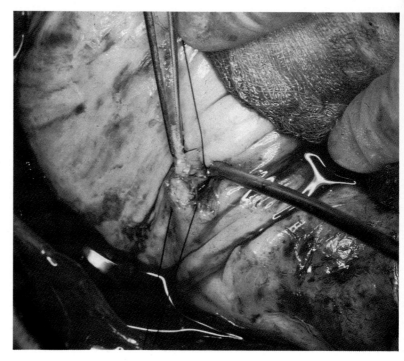

62 The right coronary artery is particularly prone to becoming blocked with extensive atheroma and, as there is often no suitable lumen for grafting, endarterectomy must be undertaken before a graft can be anastomosed. The vessel is incised longitudinally and the core of atheroma teased free.

63 A core of atheroma can then be gently pulled out. It is obviously not so important to pull out much proximally as the artery is usually blocked proximally and, anyway, a graft will be anastomosed to the arteriotomy.

64

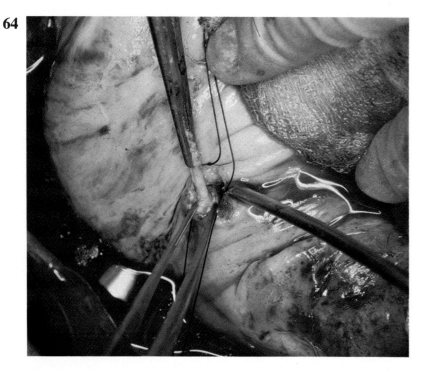

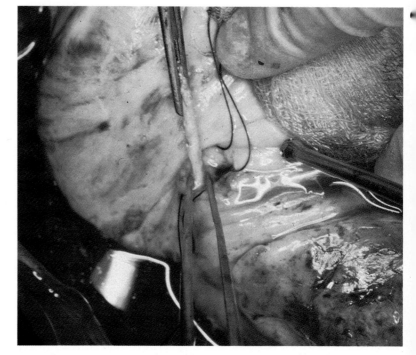

64 to 66 With careful traction, the core of atheroma is slowly removed from the distal part of the artery.

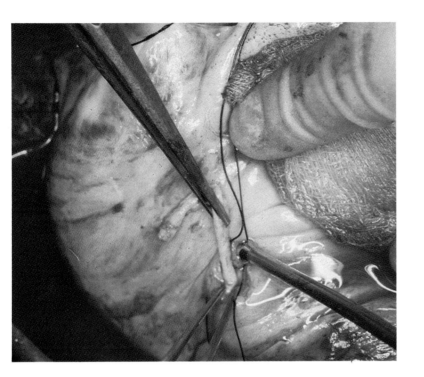
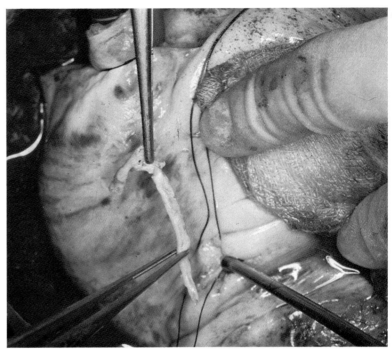

67 The atheroma, when completely removed, should show a tapering end, which indicates a smooth vessel distally.

Sequential grafts

When a patient needs many arteries grafted, sequential grafts can be used, and as this means one vein going to more than one artery, it involves side to side grafts to all but the last artery. It reduces the number of proximal anastomoses on the aorta, the length of vein needed and probably increases graft patency.

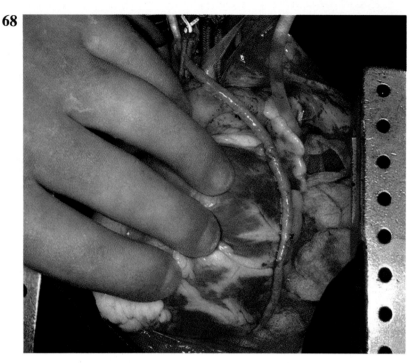

68 This sequential graft is anastomosed to three arteries.

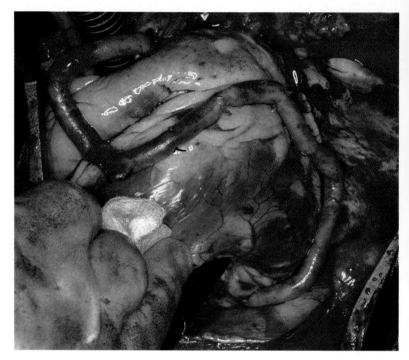

69 This vein is anastomosed to five arteries and, for obvious reasons, is sometimes called a 'snake graft'.

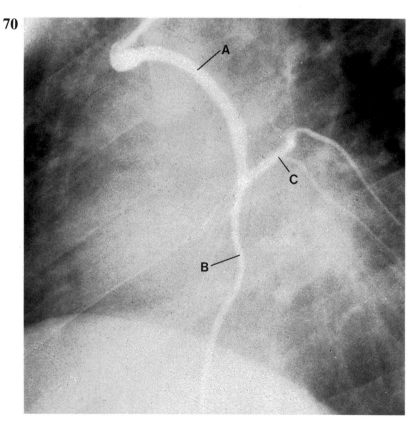

70 The post-operative angiogram shows dye filling the vein graft (**A**) and the anterior descending artery, both antegradely (**B**) and retrogradely (**C**).

10: Resection of left ventricular aneurysm

The development of a left ventricular aneurysm following myocardial infarction is quite common and the resulting left ventricular failure can be relieved by resection of the aneurysm. Careful pre-operative assessment is necessary to determine that there will be enough functioning ventricle remaining after resection. Also, there may be associated mitral regurgitation, an acquired ventricular septal defect (see Chapter 11) or coronary artery disease, any of which may need attention at the same time.

Resection of the aneurysm is carried out through the midline with the use of cardiopulmonary bypass and cold cardioplegia.

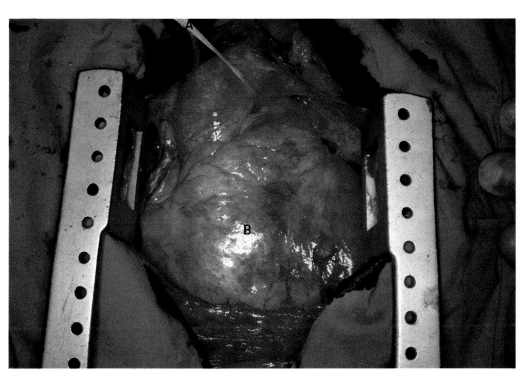

1   This view of the heart, following opening of the pericardium, shows a tape around the aorta (**A**), the prominent right ventricle (**B**) but virtually nothing of the left ventricle or aneurysm which is hidden under the left blade of the sternal retractor.

2

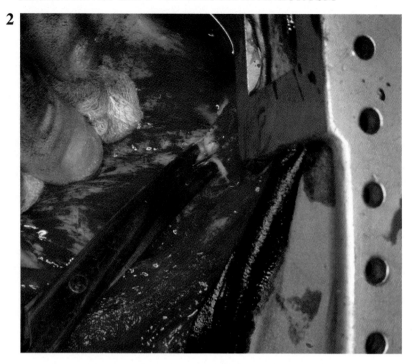

2 There are usually dense pericardial adhesions over the surface of the aneurysm and these can be seen being divided with scissors. Because of the risk of dislodging clot from inside the aneurysm, it is advisable to divide all but the anterior adhesions after the institution of cardiopulmonary bypass and clamping the aorta.

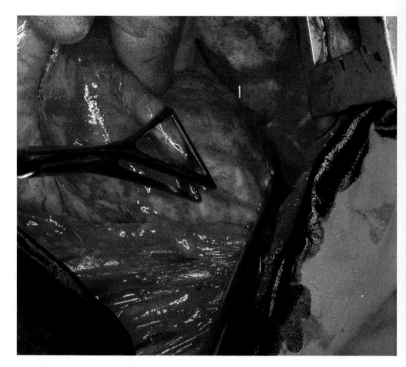

3 The heart is now empty and the collapsed wall of the aneurysm can be picked up with a Duval clamp to help further dissection of the adhesions.

4

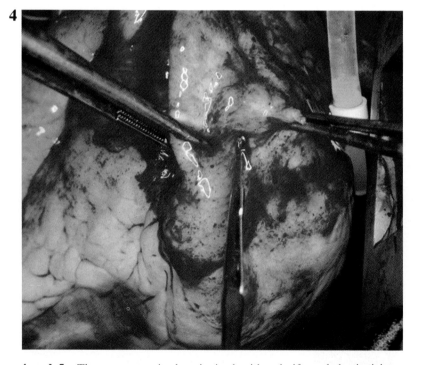

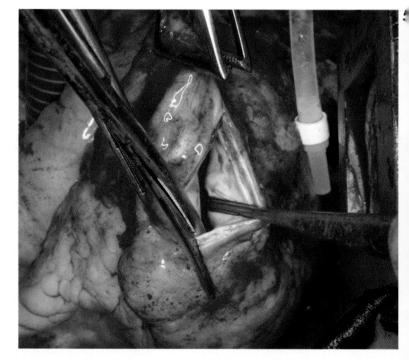

4 and 5 The aneurysm is then incised with a knife and the incision extended with scissors.

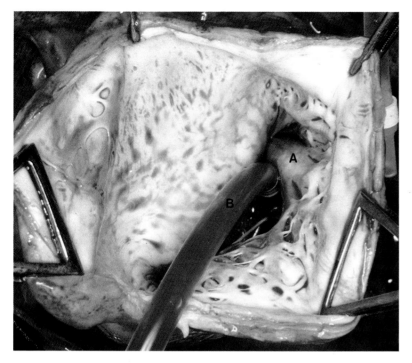

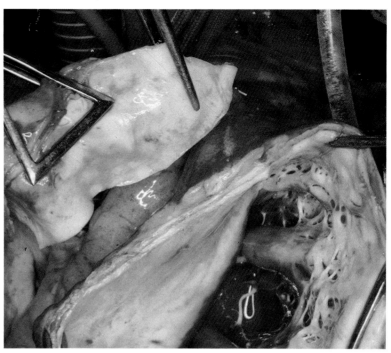

6   The fully opened aneurysm, with the walls held open by Duval clamps, shows the full extent of the aneurysm. The white fibrous lining of the aneurysm contrasts with the healthy, brown muscle of living ventricle. A papillary muscle (**A**) can be clearly seen after blood has been removed by an open suction tube (**B**).

7   The fibrous walls of the aneurysm are then removed leaving enough fibrous tissue to suture together without sacrificing any muscle. On the right side, it may not be possible to remove all the aneurysm as, in doing so, the right ventricle might be entered.

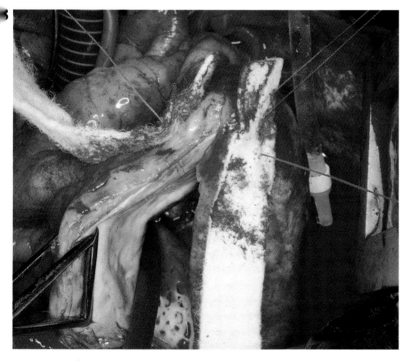

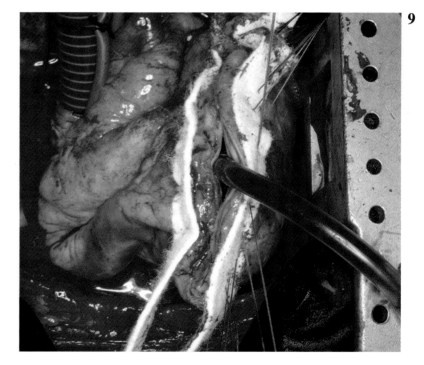

9

8 and 9   The two fibrous edges of the ventriculotomy are then approximated and firmly sutured together. It is possible to do this with a single continuous running suture, but as the ventricular tissue is sometimes rather friable, a safer method is used. This is particularly necessary as, after coming off bypass, it is often difficult even to see the ventriculotomy closure clearly, let alone repair a residual leak. The two edges are sutured together with heavy mattress sutures tied over strips of teflon felt, leaving the vent in for the present.

10

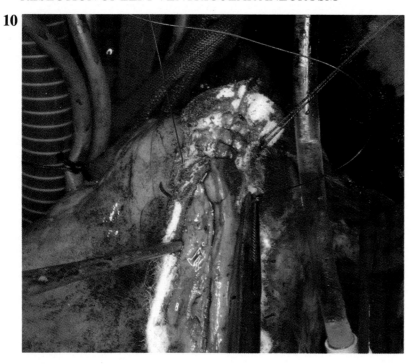

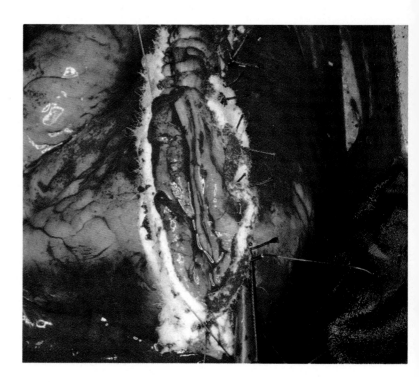

10 to 12   A continuous 2/0 Prolene suture is then run down over the incision, the vent and all air being removed after release of the aortic clamp.

12

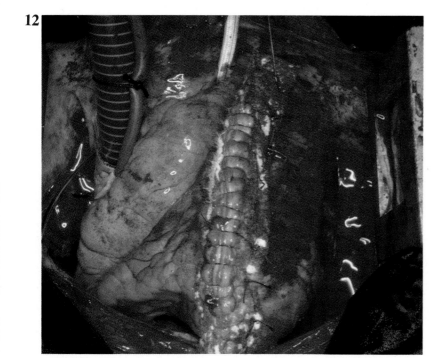

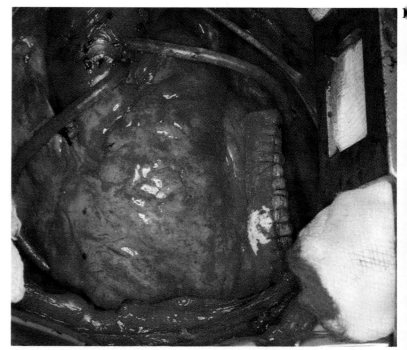

13   The final view before closing the chest shows the site of resection of the aneurysm and, in this case, two vein grafts can be seen running from the aorta to the right and circumflex coronary arteries.

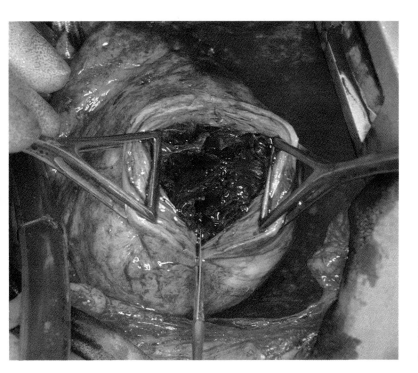

14 Sometimes when the aneurysm is incised, it is found to be full of clot. This must be carefully removed as any residual piece of clot might subsequently embolise.

11: Repair of acquired ventricular septal defect

Following myocardial infarction involving the ventricular septum, a weakness of the septum may develop and the higher pressure in the left ventricle can cause the septum to rupture. This acquired ventricular septal defect usually occurs within a few days of infarction and may quickly precipitate cardiogenic shock. Therefore, as most of these patients would die without urgent surgery, the majority present in very poor condition with ventricles that have had a recent myocardial infarction. Pre-operative assessment by angiography is neces-

sary to assess the site of the defect which can be antero-apical or posterior depending on which coronary artery was blocked. Coexisting mitral regurgitation and coronary artery disease must be assessed as these may well need attention at the same time.

Repair of the defect is carried out as for resection of the left ventricular aneurysm (see Chapter 10) but it is necessary to insert two venous cannulae and snug the cavae.

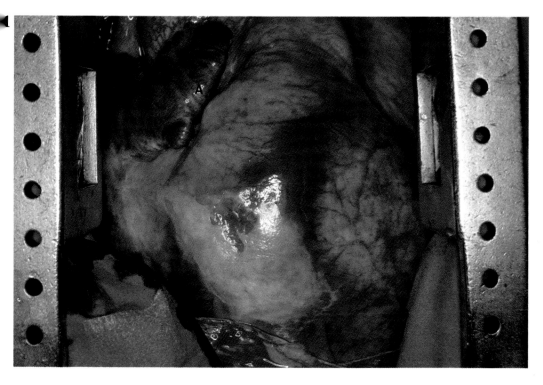

1 This view, following opening of the pericardium, shows a rather distended heart and the blood in the right atrial appendage (**A**) is very desaturated owing to the low cardiac output.

2

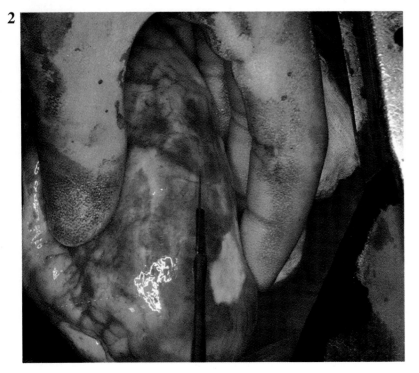

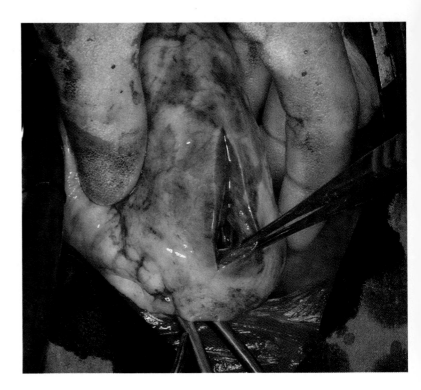

2 to 4   The apex of the left ventricle is tipped forward and the discolouration due to the recent myocardial infarction can be seen. The infarcted area is incised parallel to the anterior descending coronary artery, and the ventriculotomy cautiously retracted.

4

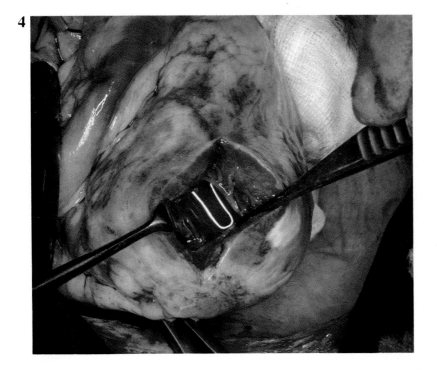

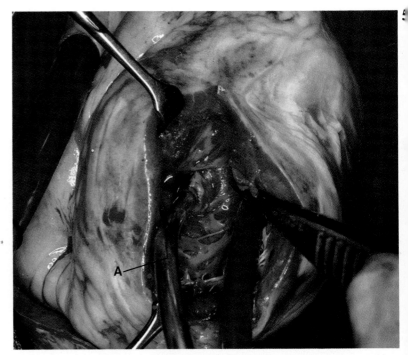

5   The incision has been enlarged and suckers positioned to remove all the blood. The metal sucker (**A**) has been passed through the ventricular septal defect and it can be clearly seen how ragged and friable the edges of the defect are.

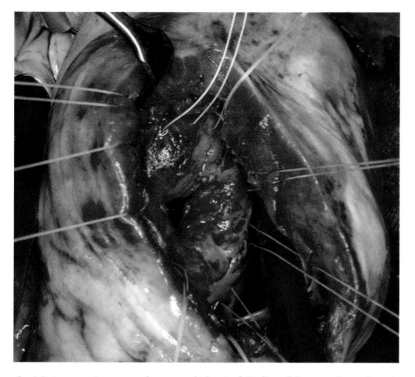

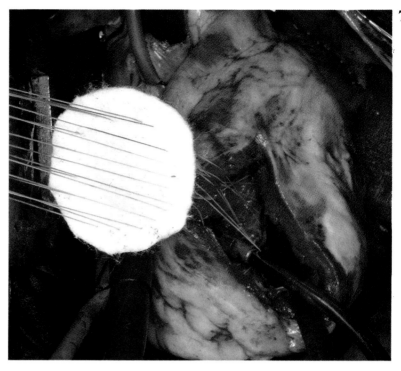

6 Mattress sutures, each on a pledget of Teflon felt, are then placed through the defect and into the muscle surrounding the defect from the right side.

7 These sutures are then placed appropriately through a large thick piece of Teflon felt.

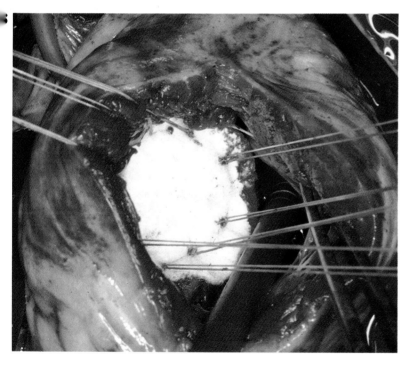

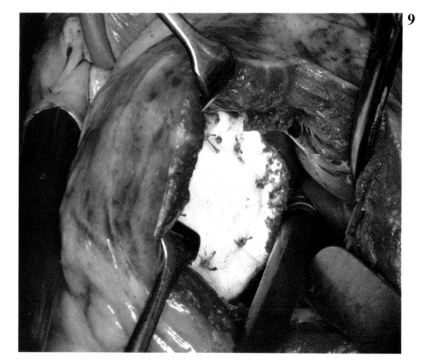

8 and 9 The Teflon felt is then tied down in position so that the septal muscle is sandwiched between the Teflon felt.

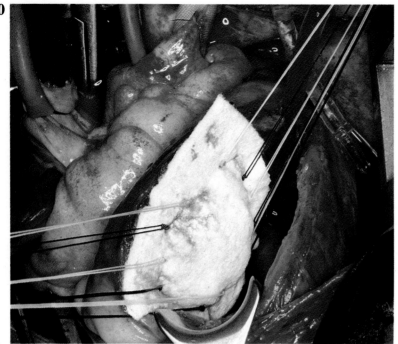 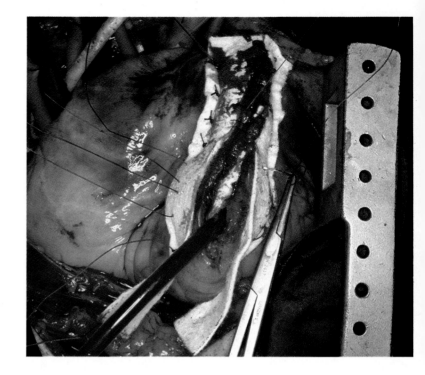

10 and 11   Sometimes, if the defect is very peripheral or the tissues unusually friable, it is better to insert a larger patch of felt and let it come out through the ventriculotomy. When the ventriculotomy is closed in the usual fashion, as for a left ventricular aneurysm (see Chapter 10), a triple deck felt and muscle sandwich is formed, providing much stronger support for the friable, necrotic ventricular muscle.

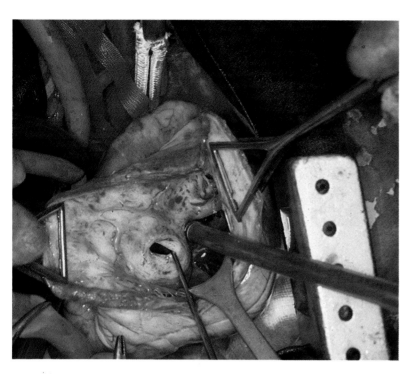

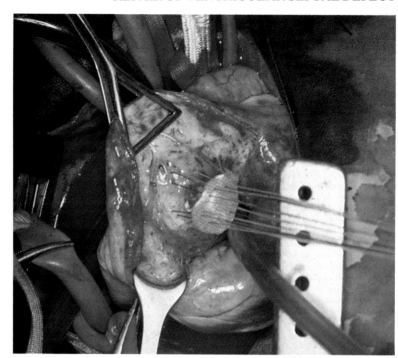

12 to 14 In some patients, the ventricular septal defect may be small and well tolerated. It therefore may be possible to wait for about six weeks after the septum has ruptured, which allows the edges of the defect to fibrose. The principles of repair are the same but, in this case, it has been possible to take smaller bites of the stronger tissue and use a Dacron patch.

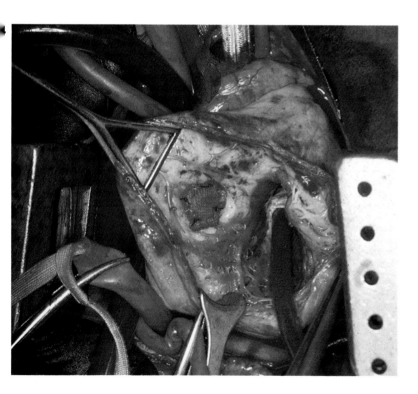

12: Replacement of ascending aorta

Replacement of the ascending aorta may be necessary in such conditions as Marfan's syndrome and medionecrosis, when the ascending aorta has become aneurysmal causing stretching of the aortic root and subsequently severe aortic regurgitation. It is necessary to replace the aortic valve and ascending aorta at the same time. Although it is sometimes possible to replace the valve separately and suture the Dacron graft above the coronary arteries, it is probably better to insert a composite graft containing a valve into the valve ring and then suture the coronary orifices direct to the graft. This avoids the risk of subsequent further stretching between the lower end of the graft and the valve ring, and was first described by Bentall and De Bono in 1968.[1]

Another reason for replacement of the ascending aorta is acute aortic dissection. This may cause aortic regurgitation because of prolapsing of the unsupported valve, and valve replacement is therefore often necessary. However, it is sometimes possible to resuspend the valve, obviating the need for replacement, and part of the ascending aorta only can be replaced, or even occasionally repaired.

Replacement of the ascending aorta is carried out through a midline sternotomy and cardiopulmonary bypass is used. As the aortic clamp must be placed as far distal on the ascending aorta as possible, it is usual to cannulate the femoral artery for the arterial return from the cardiopulmonary bypass machine. The venous return can be taken from the right atrium as for aortic valve replacement. Perfusion of the coronary arteries with cardioplegic solution is most helpful, although the operation can be performed with coronary artery perfusion.

Cannulation of femoral artery

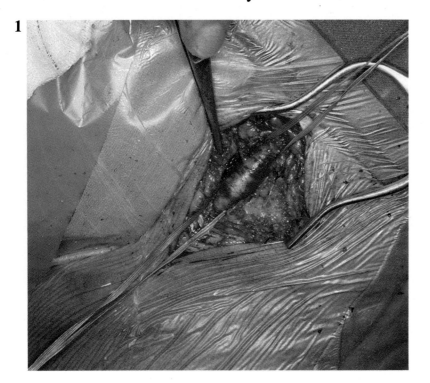

1 The femoral artery is exposed and taped.

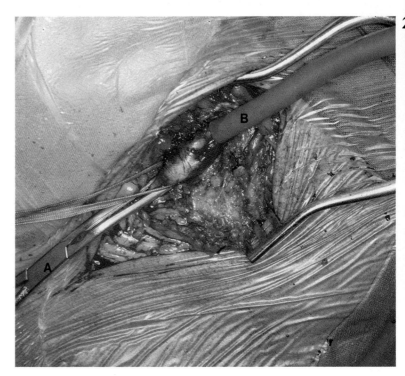

2 A clamp is applied below (**A**) and a tape snugged down on a rubber tube above (**B**).

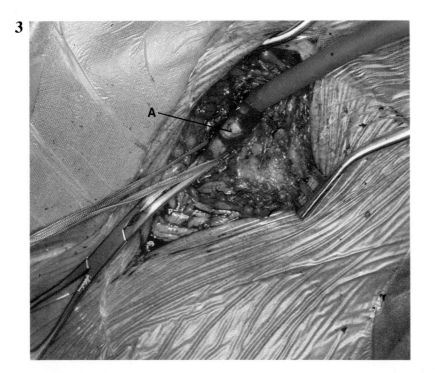

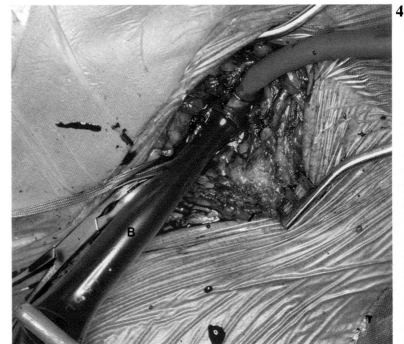

3 and 4 A transverse incision (**A**) is made in the artery and a cannula (**B**) is inserted. The rubber is released to allow insertion of the cannula and then snugged again to prevent a leak.

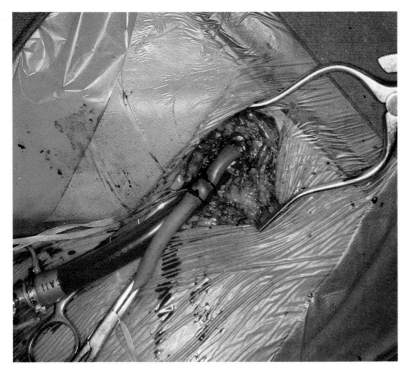

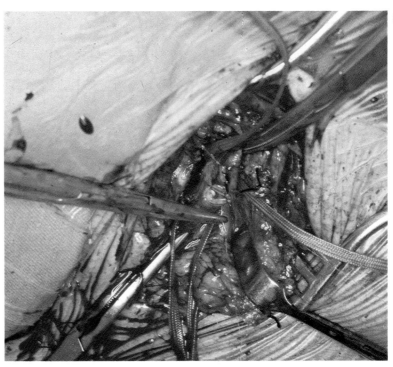

5 The cannula is firmly tied to the rubber snugger to prevent dislodgement during bypass.

6 and 7 After bypass has been discontinued, the cannula is removed, the arteriotomy sutured and the clamps released.

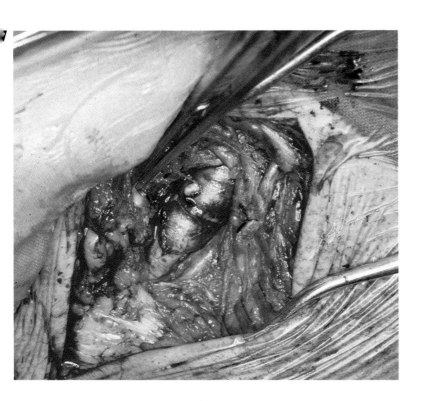

Replacement of ascending aorta

8

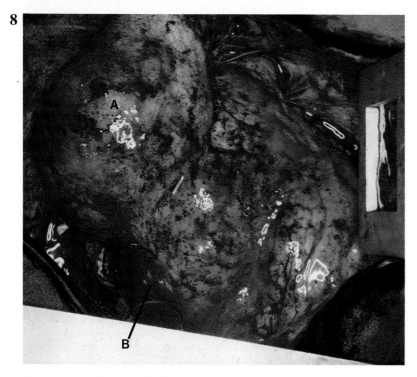

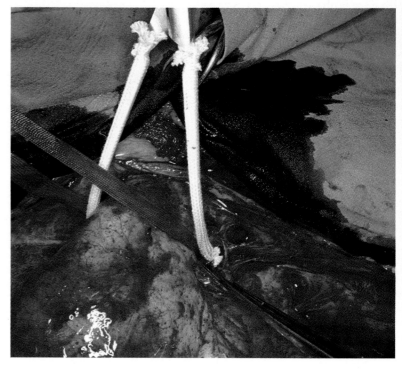

8   The ascending aorta (**A**) is grossly aneurysmal. The venous cannula (**B**) can be seen coming from the atrial appendage.

9   Bypass has been commenced and the ascending aorta is about to be clamped.

10

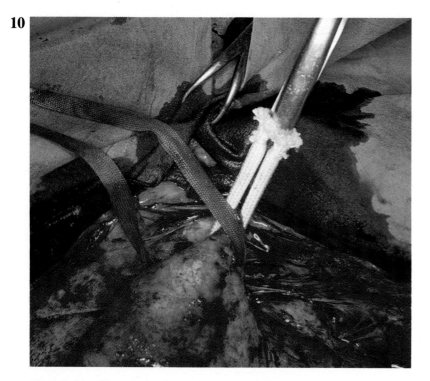

1

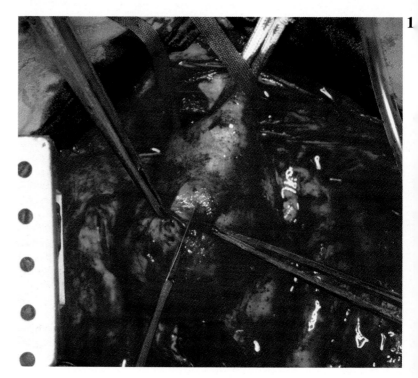

10 and 11   The aortic clamp has been applied just proximal to the innominate artery and the aorta is about to be incised.

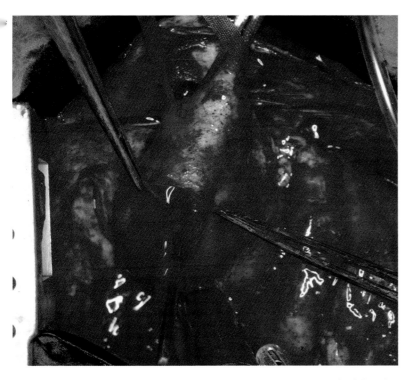

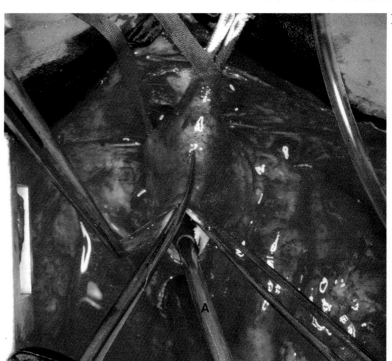

12 and 13 The aorta has been incised with a knife and the incision is extended upwards with scissors. A sucker (**A**) is used to return blood to the cardiopulmonary bypass machine.

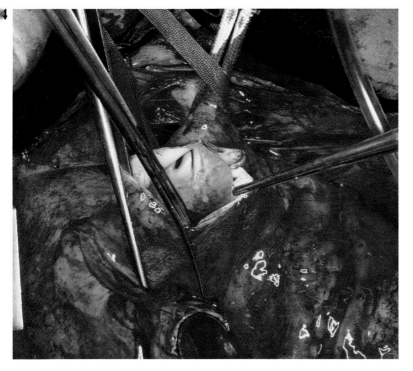

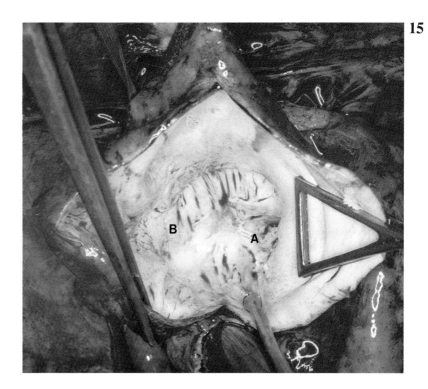

14 and 15 The incision is extended downwards and the enormously dilated aortic root displayed. The valve (**A**) can just be seen and a large thin-walled area of aorta (**B**) occupies much of the remainder of the aortic root.

16

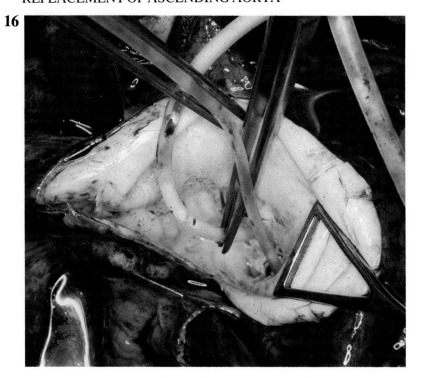

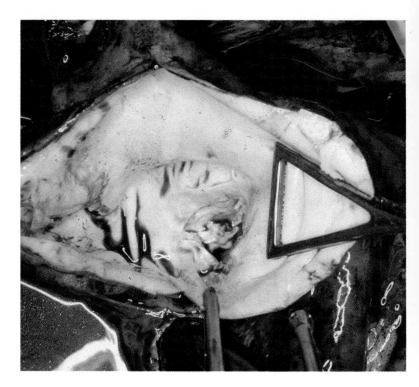

16 to 18 . Cardioplegic solution is perfused into the coronary arteries. The aortic valve has been excised and the size of the aortic root is measured.

18

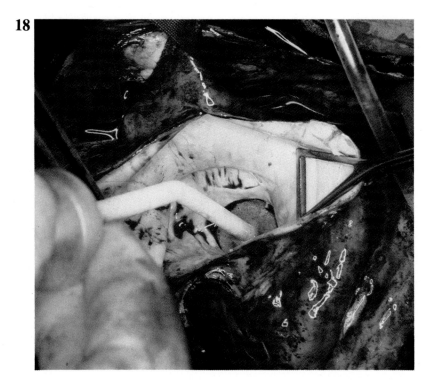

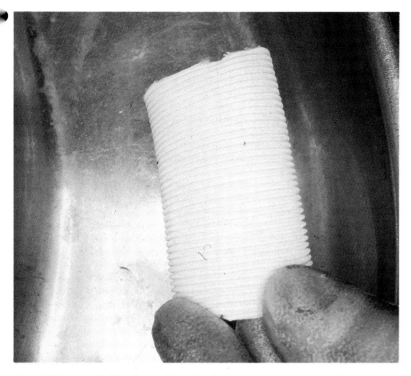

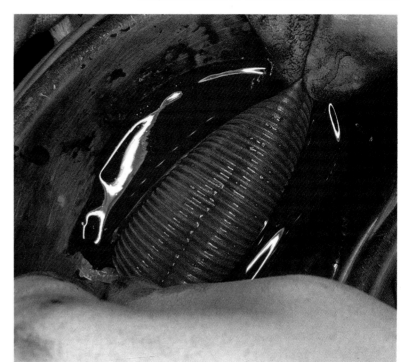

19 and 20 A suitable size and length of woven Dacron tube is selected and preclotted by soaking it in some of the patient's unheparinised blood. This preclotting helps to fill the interstices of the graft with clot and therefore minimises bleeding later.

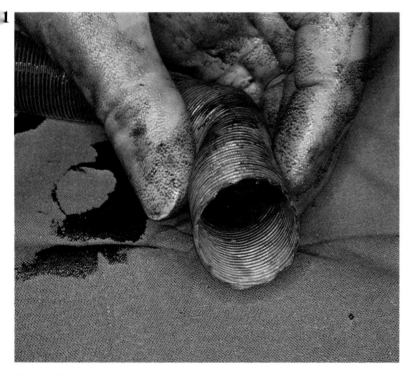

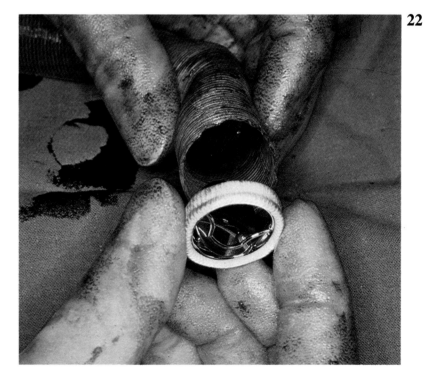

21 and 22 Any type of valve can be sewn into the Dacron tube but a low-profile valve, such as the Bjork–Shiley, makes for easier insertion of the graft. A suitable size of valve is selected for the size of the graft.

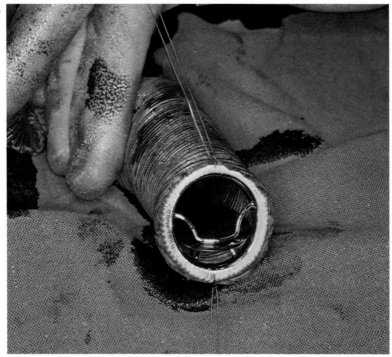

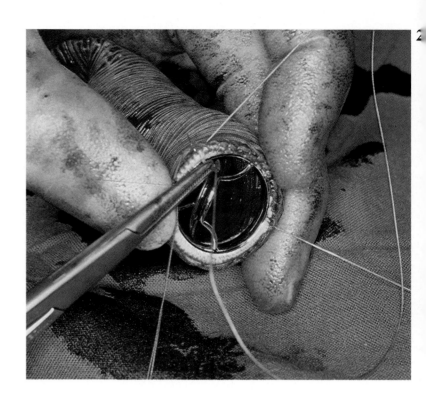

23 to 25 The valve is then sutured into the end of the tube with a continuous suture. Some ready-made composite grafts with valves *in situ* are available, but tend to leak through the graft.

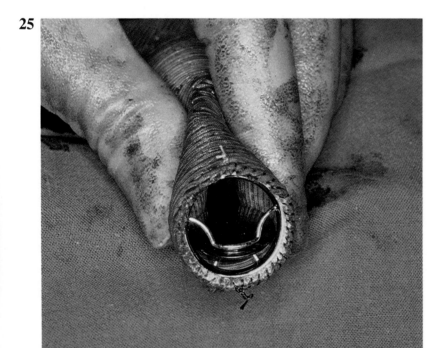

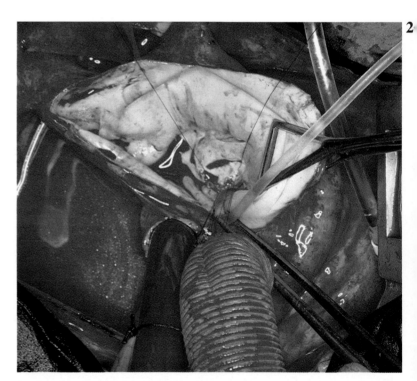

26 The composite graft is then sutured down into the aortic root using a continuous Prolene suture. Here several sutures have been placed before sliding the valve down.

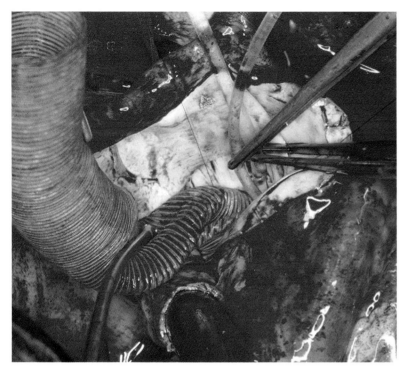

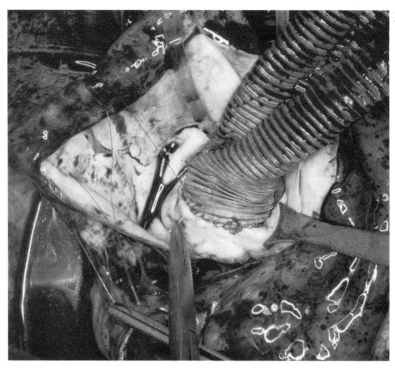

27 As the coronary orifices are above the aortic root to which the graft has been sutured, it is possible to give more cardioplegic solution if necessary, as in this case.

28 The continuous suture can be seen coming up the right side of the anastomosis.

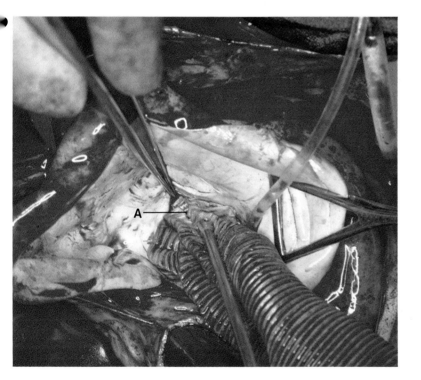

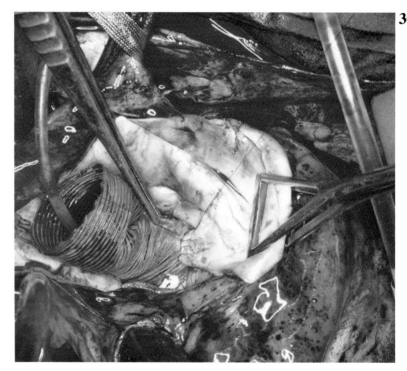

29 A hole (**A**) has been cut in the graft to attach the left coronary orifice and this is then sutured with a continuous suture around the left coronary orifice.

30 The right coronary orifice has been similarly anastomosed to a suitably placed hole in the graft, and the continuous suture is just about to be tied.

31
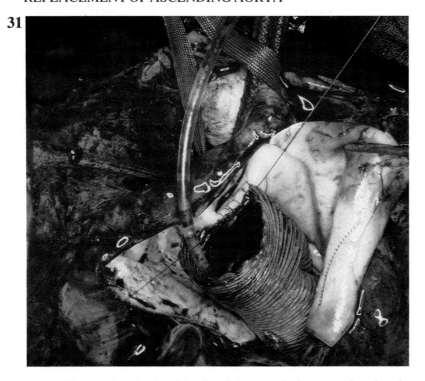

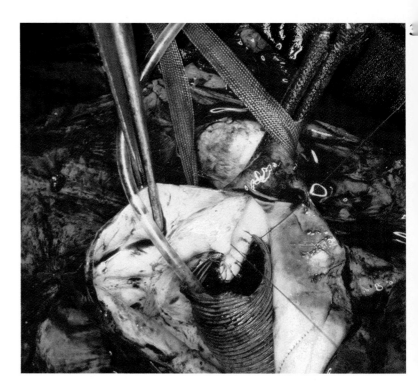

31 and 32 The length of graft is trimmed to exactly the correct length and the upper anastomosis is performed starting posteriorly.

33
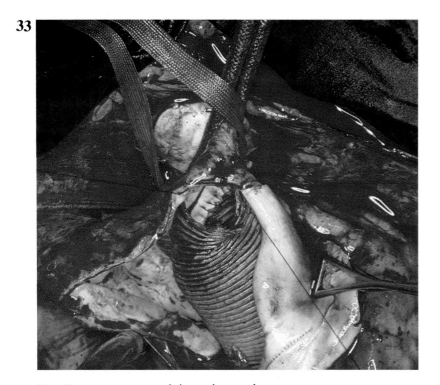

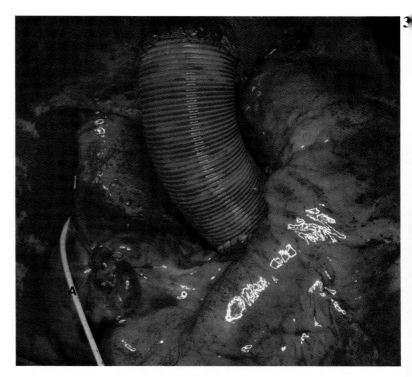

33 The upper anastomosis is nearly complete.

34 Bypass has been discontinued and the final appearance of the graft seen before closing the chest. The white catheter (**A**) is a left atrial pressure line.

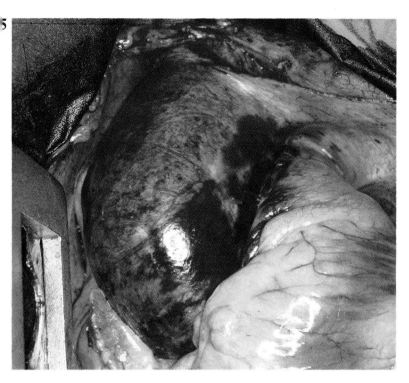

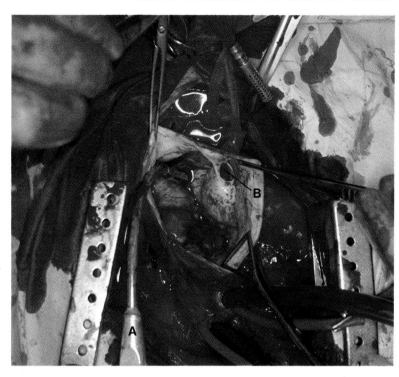

35 This pre-operative picture, in another patient, shows the typical appearance in acute dissection of the aorta.

36 The appearance of a dissection once the aorta is open is shown here. The sucker (**A**) is in the false lumen, and the communication (**B**) with the true lumen can be seen.

13: Replacement of descending aorta

Replacement of part of the descending aorta may be required for an aneurysm, dissection or acute rupture. Aneurysms are most commonly situated just distal to the subclavian artery and may be degenerative in origin, or follow previous dissection or, rarely, rupture. As the aorta must be clamped above and below the aneurysm for its removal, the spinal cord and lower parts of the body should be protected by femoral artery perfusion (see Chapter 12). Blood may be taken from the left atrium, femoral vein or pulmonary artery for the return to the cardiopulmonary bypass machine. It is also possible to use a direct shunt from the left ventricle to the descending aorta or femoral artery and this may be particularly useful in the case of a ruptured aorta following trauma.

Aneurysms of the aorta are often very large and are not very photogenic. If they have already ruptured, the technical difficulty and risk of the procedure are considerably increased. The approach is through a left thoracotomy and the level depends on the level of the aneurysm, but for most aneurysms that are situated just distal to the left subclavian artery, the fourth intercostal space is satisfactory (see Chapter 3).

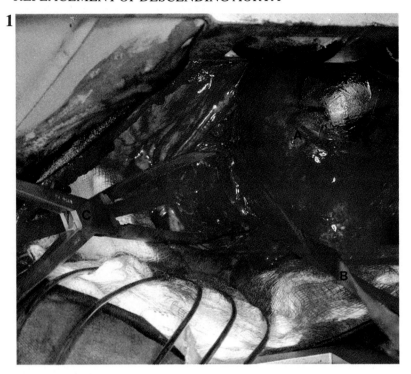

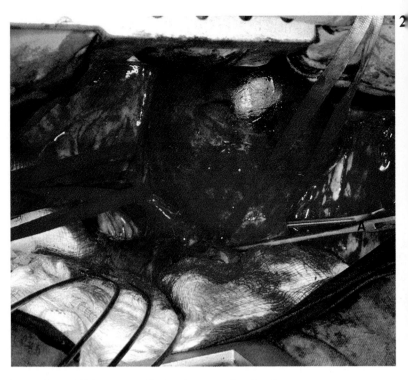

1   The aneurysm (**A**) has been dissected from the lung and a tape (**B**) passed around the aortic arch. A clamp (**C**) is being applied to the aortic arch proximal to the aneurysm.

2   A clamp (**A**) is now applied to the aorta distal to the aneurysm.

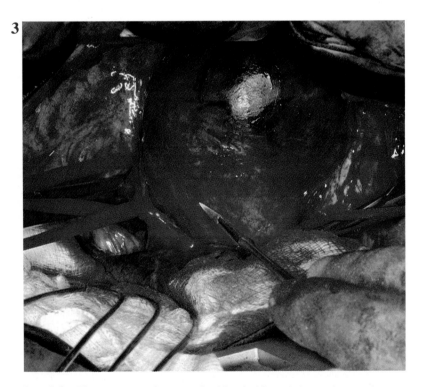

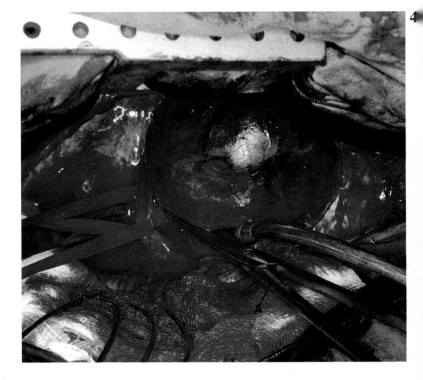

3 and 4   The aneurysm is opened with a knife and then scissors (**A**). A sucker removes blood, which is returned to the cardiopulmonary bypass machine.

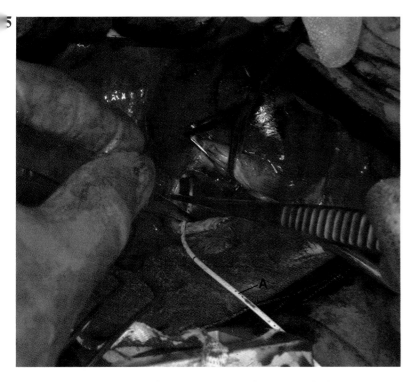

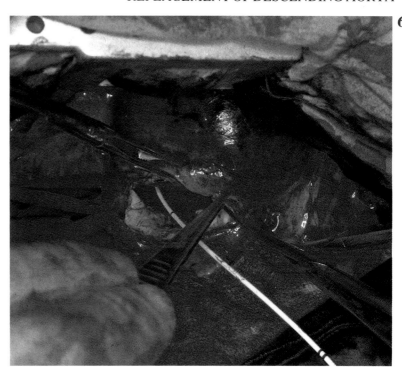

5 and 6   In this case, the left subclavian artery is involved in the aneurysm. However, as it cannot be clamped because of poor access, a Fogarty catheter (**A**) has been inserted into it and inflation of the balloon used to occlude it.

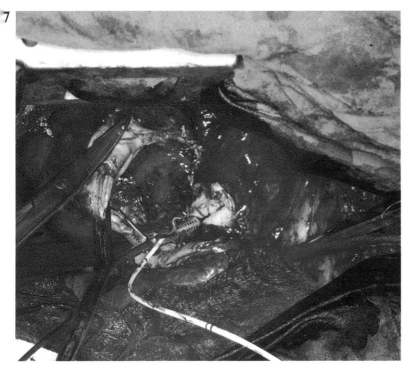

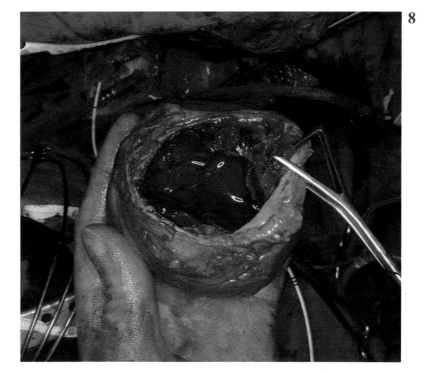

7 and 8   The aneurysm in this area has been completely excised and is full of thrombus.

9

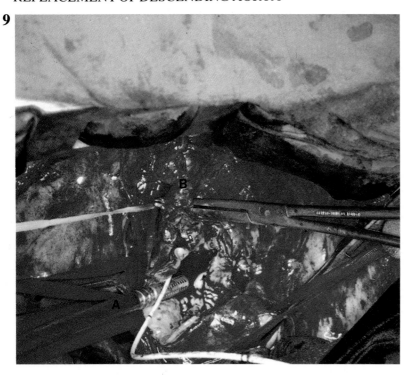

1

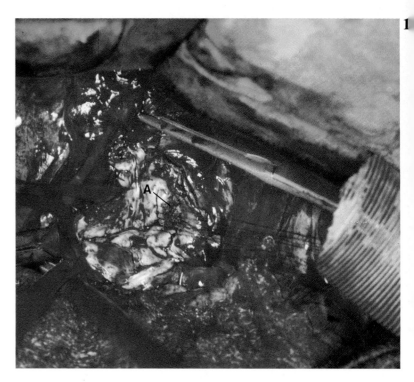

9   A sucker (**A**) returns blood to the bypass machine and the subclavian artery (**B**) is clamped and the Fogarty cannula removed.

10   A preclotted woven Dacron tube graft is then sutured to the proximal aorta. Here the Prolene suture has been placed through the graft and aorta several times before sliding the graft down into position. A piece of Teflon felt (**A**) has been used to support the sutures in the weak aortic tissue posteriorly.

11

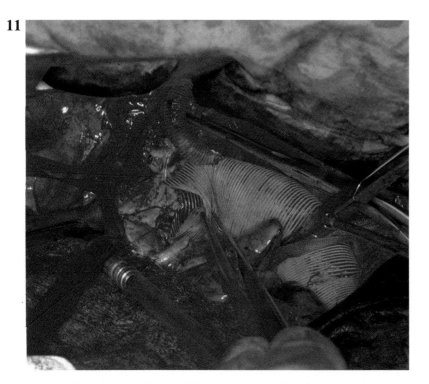

1

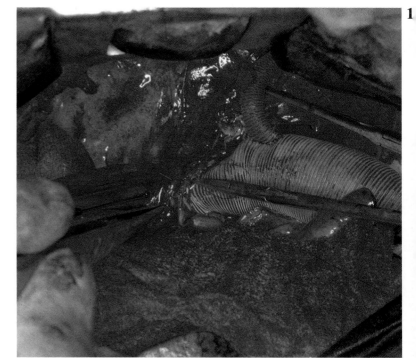

11 and 12   The remainder of the upper suture line is completed with continuous Prolene.

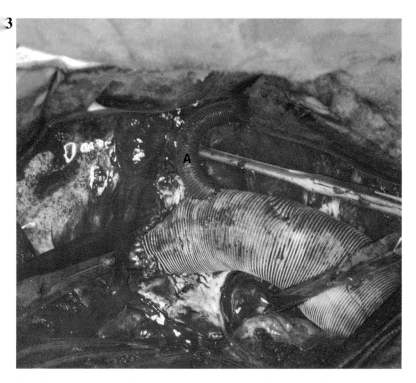

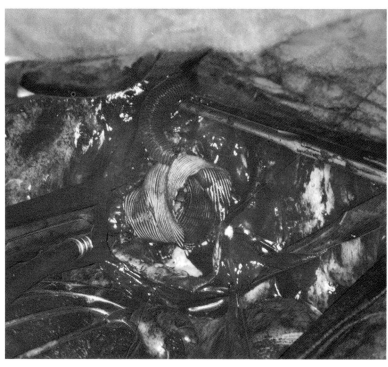

13 The upper suture line has been completed and the graft clearly seen. A side arm (**A**) has been sutured to it in this case, for later attachment of the subclavian artery.

14 The graft is cut to the required length, and the lower anastomosis performed, again with a continuous suture.

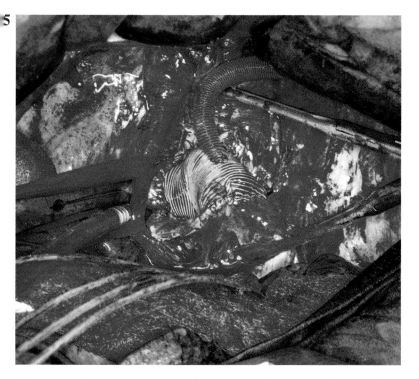

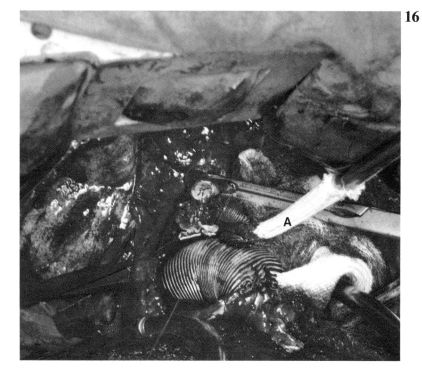

15 and 16 The lower anastomosis has been completed and, after clamping the side arm graft with a soft clamp (**A**), the aortic clamps can be released.

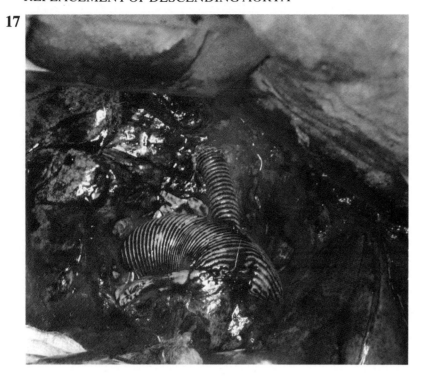

17 The side arm has now been anastomosed to the left subclavian artery and the resection is complete.

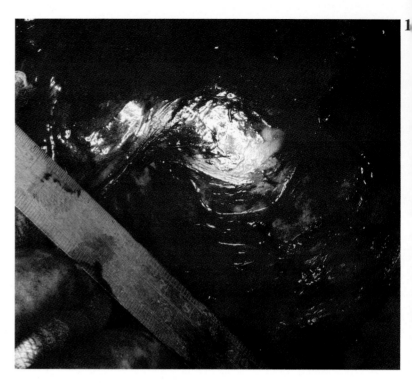

18 This is a massive descending aortic aneurysm in a different patient, measuring at least 10 cm.

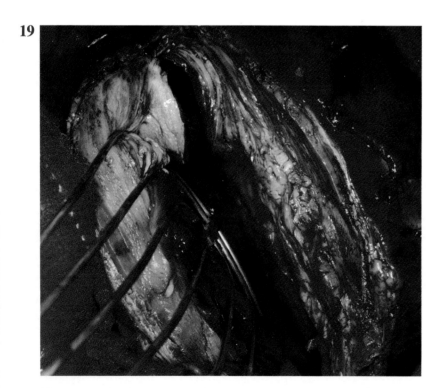

19 On opening the aneurysm, there is a very thick layer of laminated clot.

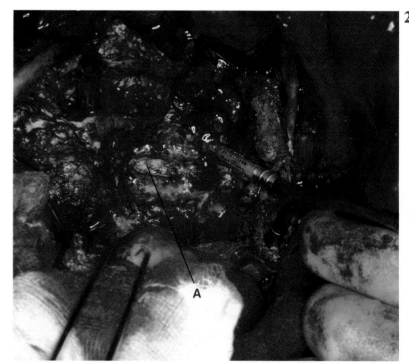

20 It can be seen that the base of the aneurysm is, in fact, formed by the spinal column, the bone of which has been eroded by the aneurysm. However, one of the cartilaginous intervertebral discs (**A**) can be seen and is less eroded.

14: Removal of atrial myxoma

Myxomas, although rare, are the most frequently encountered tumours of the heart and, although they can occur in any chamber, are usually found in the left atrium. Diagnosis can be extremely difficult but two-dimensional echocardiography is very helpful. These tumours are often rather friable, having a gelatinous nature, and they may embolise. They may, in fact, be diagnosed by the removal of myxoma tissue at embolectomy and great care must be taken in handling them at operation.

In approaching a left atrial myxoma, it is usually best to go through the right atrium and make a 'Dubost' incision into the left atrium and incise the atrial septum. This gives a wider orifice through which the myxoma may be 'delivered'. The myxoma is usually attached by a short, wide pedicle to the atrial septum and this, together with its surrounding tissue, should be removed at operation. Although these tumours only recur very rarely, it is important to remove the site of attachment to minimise the possibility. The defect in the atrial septum caused by the removal of the pedicle can be closed with a patch.

Obviously cardiopulmonary bypass is used and two venous cannulae must be inserted and the cavae snugged to allow opening of the right atrium.

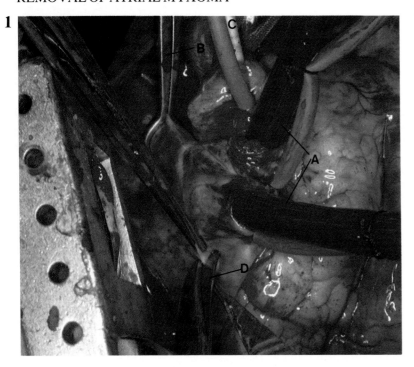

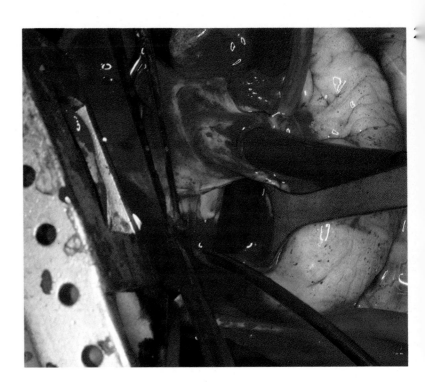

1 and 2 Cannulae (**A**) have been inserted into the venae cavae and the cavae snugged. (In this case they have been snugged with Cooley caval clamps (**B**).) The aorta has been clamped and cardioplegic solution infused through a cannula (**C**) into the ascending aorta. The right atrium is then incised with scissors (**D**) and retracted.

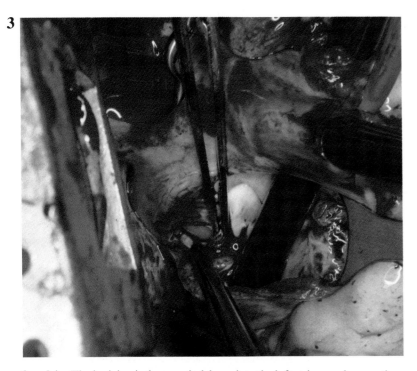

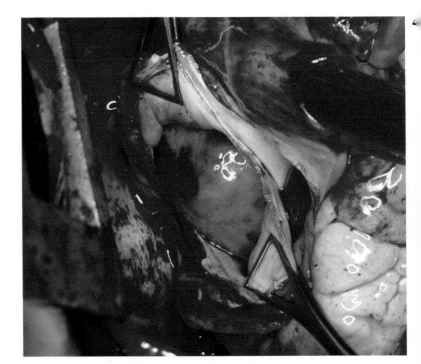

3 and 4 The incision is then carried down into the left atrium and across the atrial septum to reveal the glistening myxoma in the left atrium.

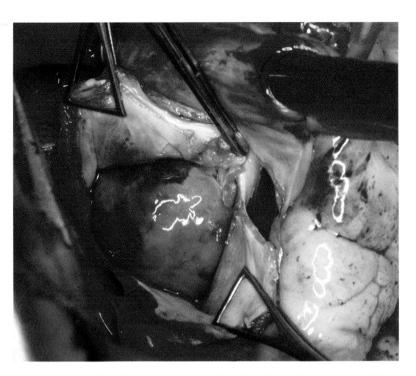
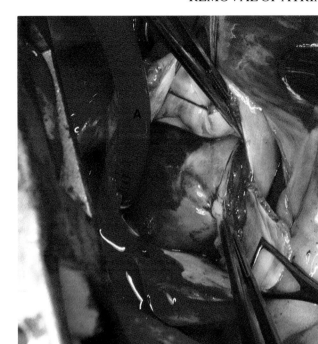

5 to 8 The incision is extended to the far side of the atrial septum and the pedicle carefully dissected away. Care must be taken not to dissect too deeply as the pedicle can be attached close to the root of the aorta – as in this case. An atrial suction vent (**A**) has been inserted to remove blood returning to the left atrium.

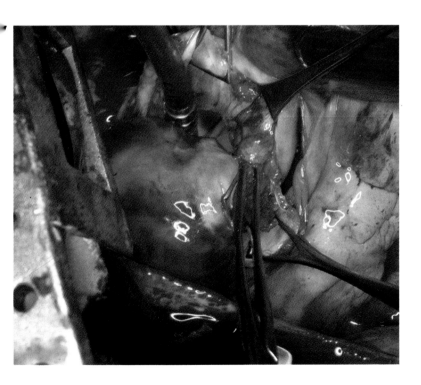
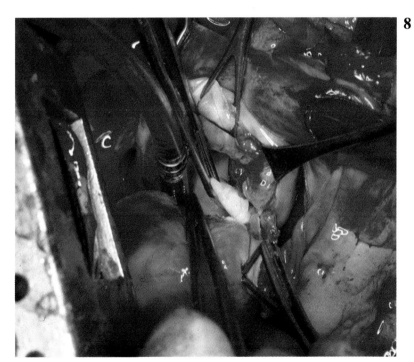

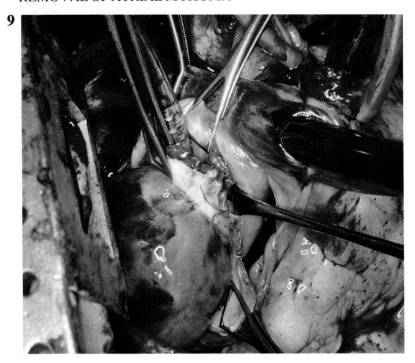

9

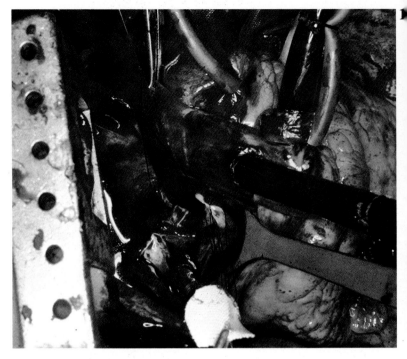

9 The pedicle has now been completely freed and the myxoma is carefully lifted from the heart.

10 to 12 The defect in the atrial septum is then closed with a Dacron patch, air removed from the left side of the heart and the right atrium closed.

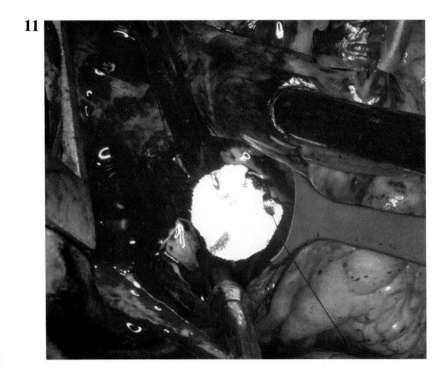

11

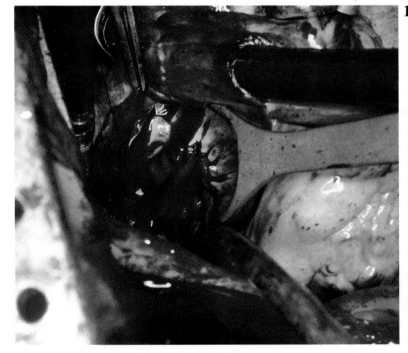

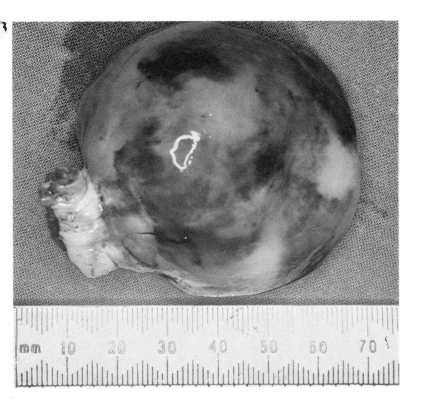

13 The myxoma excised in this case is seen to be about 6 cm in diameter.

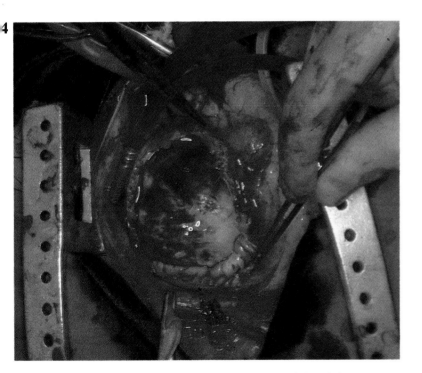

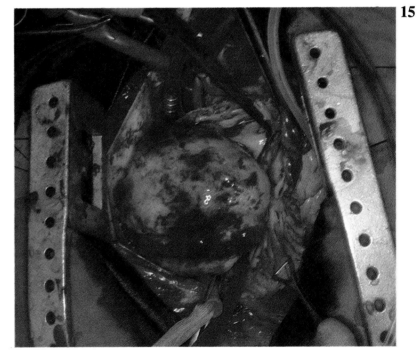

14 and 15 These pictures show the removal of a huge right atrial myxoma. Cannulation of the cavae can be very difficult, and it may be necessary to cannulate the cavae directly.

15: Pericardiectomy

Pericardiectomy is required for symptomatic constrictive pericarditis. The aetiology of the chronic pericardial constriction is often unknown, but tuberculosis should certainly be sought for and often treated speculatively. For removal of the constriction, the heart may be approached either through a midline sternotomy or by a bilateral sub-mammary approach. It is rarely necessary to use cardiopulmonary bypass. The pericardium is usually thickened to about 3 mm and may contain fluid, caseous material and altered blood. Though the removal of the pericardium itself may greatly relieve the constriction, the epicardium of the heart also becomes thickened and constricts the heart, and this layer should also be removed. It is usually stuck firmly to the surface of the heart and care must be taken in removing it, not to damage the coronary arteries. However, despite great care, this operation can often be extremely haemorrhagic.

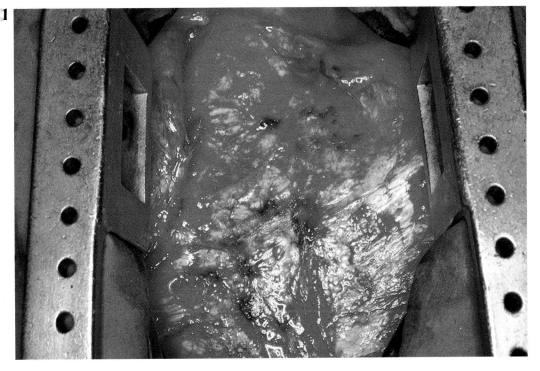

1 The sternum has been split and the thickened, haemorrhagic pericardium is seen before opening.

2

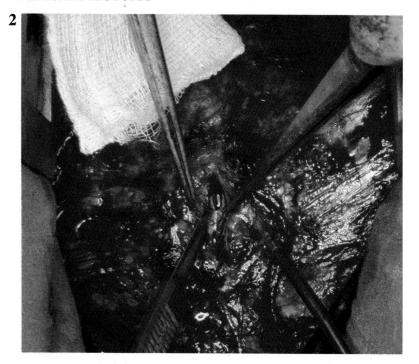

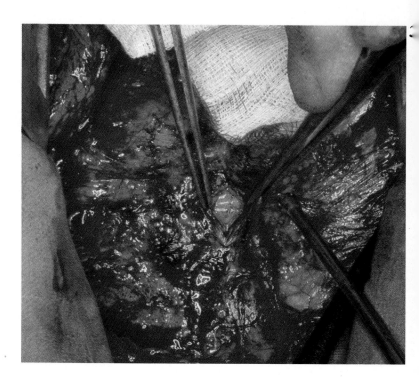

2 and 3   A knife is used to cautiously incise the pericardium and expose the heart, which can be seen covered by thick, white epicardium.

4

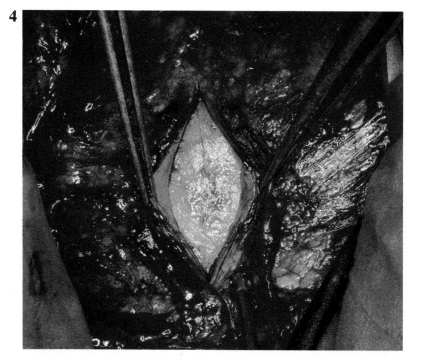

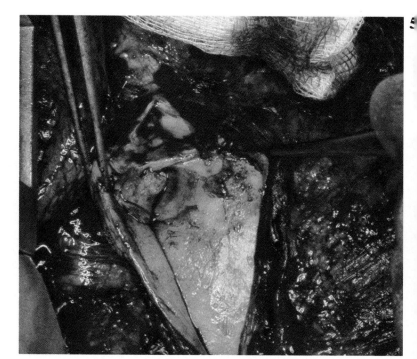

4 and 5   The pericardium is incised with scissors and with careful dissection it can be freed from the heart completely.

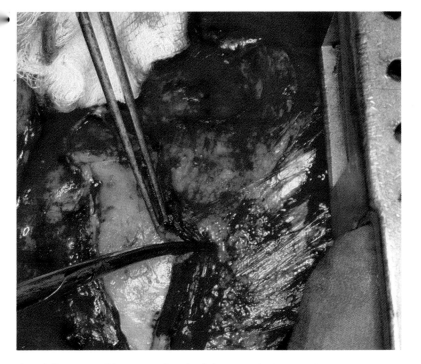

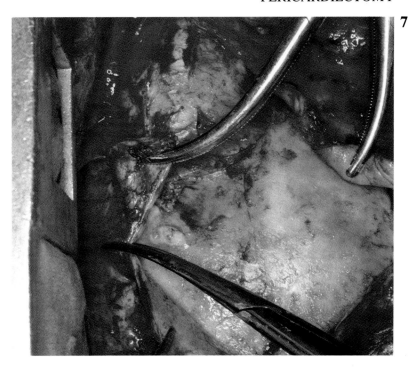

6 and 7 By making a cruciate incision anteriorly, careful dissection of each quarter of pericardium can be achieved, allowing the heart to bulge out anteriorly from its constriction.

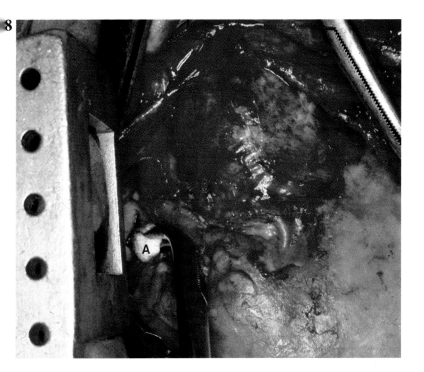

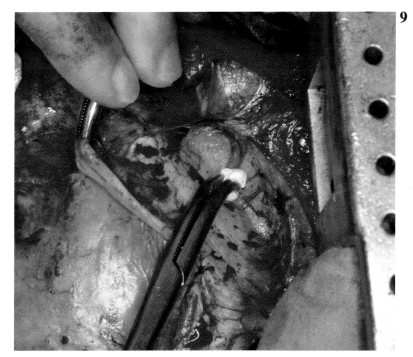

8 A Lahey swab (**A**) may be used for blunt dissection, but great care should be taken around the right atrium, as the atrial wall may be extremely thin and as the right atrial pressure is usually very high, even a small tear can give rise to desperate bleeding.

9 Here, blunt dissection is being used to dissect the lung from the pericardium, so that a large piece of pericardium can be removed, without opening the pleura.

10

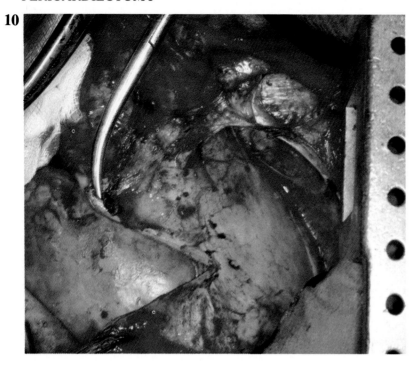

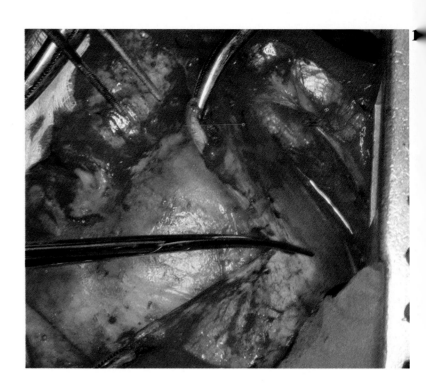

10 and 11 The left lateral incision into the pericardium is then continued, but care must be taken not to go so far posteriorly that the phrenic nerve is damaged.

12

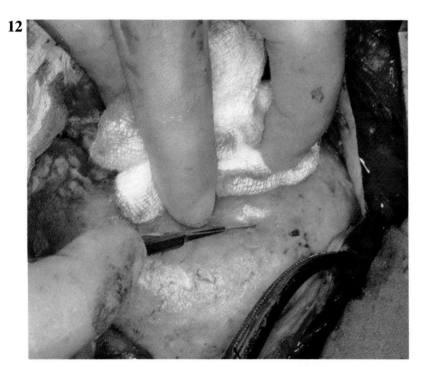

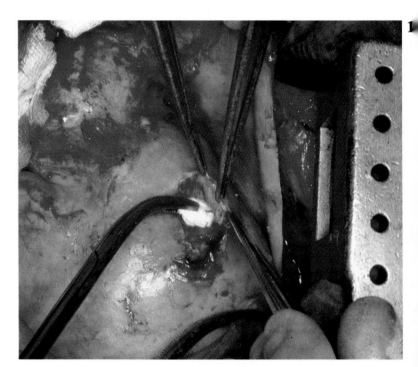

12 and 13 A further cruciate incision is made in the thickened epicardium, which overlies the heart itself. The dissection is then continued in each direction.

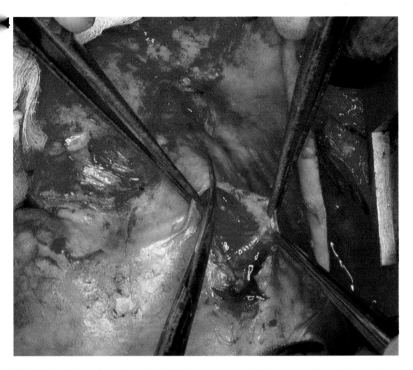

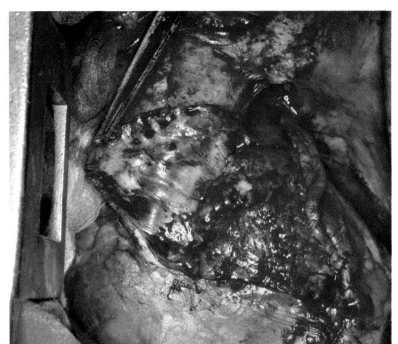

14 to 17 The epicardium having been removed, the unrestricted, but rather haemorrhagic, heart is revealed.

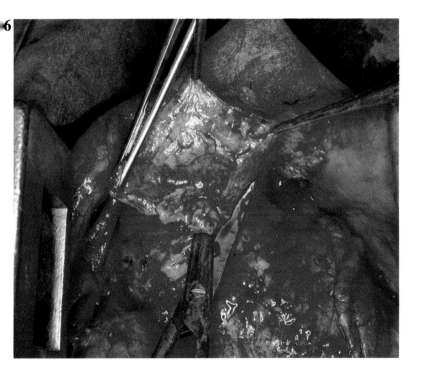

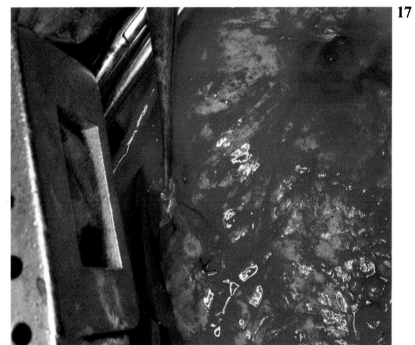

18

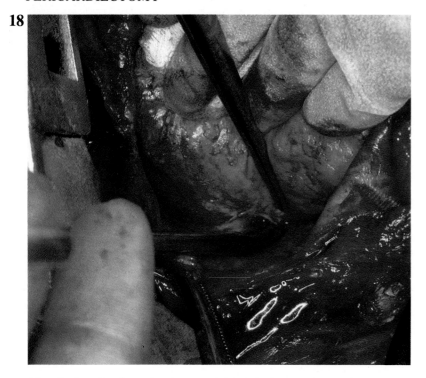

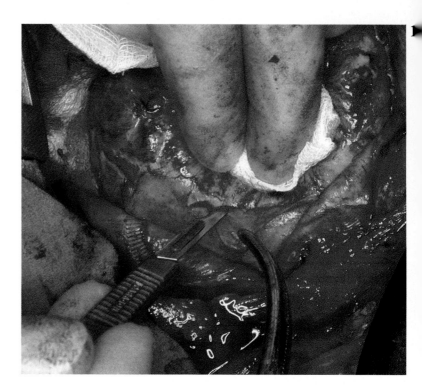

18 and 19 The dissection is extended inferiorly to free the inferior vena cava.

20

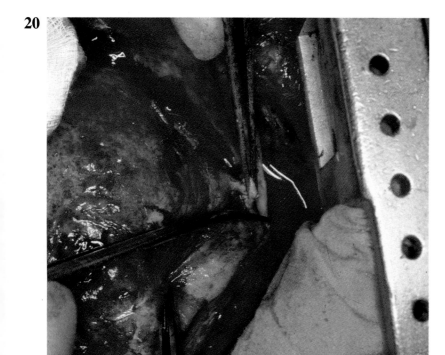

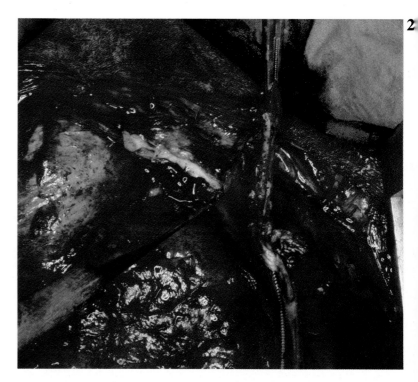

20 The dissection is continued towards the apex.

21 The excess pericardium is removed, and this can be conveniently done with diathermy as the pericardium is usually very haemorrhagic.

References

Chapter 1

1   Manners J. M. (1980) Anaesthesia for cardiac surgery. In *Topical reviews in Anaesthesia*. Ed: J. Norman & J. Whitwam, Vol. 1, pp.179–260. Wright, Bristol.
2   Ionescu M. I. (1981) *Techniques in Extracorporeal Circulation*. Butterworths, Sevenoaks.
3   Roe B.B., Hutchinson J. C., Fishman N. H., Ullyot D.J. and Smith D.L. (1977) Myocardial protection with cold, ischaemic, potassium-induced cardioplegia. *Journal of Thoracic and Cardiovascular Surgery* **73**, 366.
4   Harris E.A., Neutze J.M., Rickard M. P., Seelye E.R. and Simpson M. M. (1975) *Intensive Care of the Heart and Lungs*. Blackwell Scientific Publications, Oxford and London.

Chapter 4

1   Harken D.E., Soroff H.S., Taylor W.J., Lefemire A.A. and Lunzer S. (1960) Partial and complete prosthesis in aortic insufficiency. *Journal of Thoracic and Cardiovascular Surgery* **40**, 744.
2   Starr A., Edwards M.L., McCord C.W. and Griswold H.E. (1963) Aortic replacement. Clinical experience with a semi-rigid ball-valve prosthesis. *Circulation* **27**, 779.
3   Bjork V.O., Henze A. and Holmgren A. (1974) Five years' experience with the Bjork–Shiley tilting disc valve in isolated aortic valvular disease. *Journal of Thoracic and Cardiovascular Surgery* **68**, 393.
4   Ross D. N. (1962) Homograft replacement of the aortic valve. *Lancet* **ii**, 487.
5   Barratt-Boyes B.G. (1964) Homograft aortic valve replacement in aortic incompetence and stenosis *Thorax* **19**, 131.
6   Khanna S. K., Ross J. K. and Monro J.L. (1981) Homograft aortic valve replacement: seven years' experience with antibiotic-treated valves. *Thorax* **36**, 330.
7   Barratt-Boyes B.G. (1965) Method for preparing and inserting a homograft valve. *British Journal of Surgery* **52**, 847.

Chapter 5

1   Cutler E.C. and Levine S.A. (1923) Cardiotomy and valvulotomy for mitral stenosis. Experimental observations and clinical notes concerning an operated case with recovery. *Boston M. & S. Journal* **188**, 1023.
2   Carpentier A., Deloche A., Dauptain J., Soyer R., Blondeau P., Piwnica A. and Dubost C. (1971) A new reconstructive operation for correction of mitral and tricuspid insufficiency. *Journal of Thoracic and Cardiovascular Surgery* **61**, 1.

Chapter 6

1   Bjork V.O. and Henze A. (1979) A ten years' experience with the Bjork–Shiley tilting disc valve. *Journal of Thoracic and Cardiovascular Surgery* **78**, 331.
2   Oyer P. E., Stinson E. B., Reitz B.A., Miller D.C., Rossiter S.J. and Shumway N. E. (1979) Long-term evaluation of the porcine xenograft bioprosthesis. *Journal of Thoracic and Cardiovascular Surgery* **78**, 343.

Chapter 7

1   Carpentier A., Deloche A., Dauptain J., Soyer R., Blondeau P., Piwnica A. and Dubost C. (1971) A new reconstructive operation for correction of mitral and tricuspid insufficiency. *Journal of Thoracic and Cardiovascular Surgery* **61**, 1.
2   De Vega N.G. (1972) La annuloplastia selectiva, regulable y permanente. *Rev. Esp. Cardiol.* **25**, 6.
3   Grondin P., Meere C., Limet R., Lopez-Bescos L., Delcan J-L. and Rivera R. (1975) Carpentier's annulus and De Vega's annuloplasty. *Journal of Thoracic and Cardiovascular Surgery* **70**, 852.

Chapter 8

1   Bourdillon P. V. D. and Sharratt G. P. (1976) Malfunction of Bjork–Shiley prosthesis in tricuspid position. *British Heart Journal* **38**, 1149.

Chapter 9

1   Favoloro R. G. (1969) Saphenous vein graft in the surgical treatment of coronary artery disease. *Journal of Thoracic and Cardiovascular Surgery* **58**, 178.

Chapter 12

1   Bentall H. and De Bono A. (1968) A technique for complete replacement of the ascending aorta. *Thorax* **23**, 338.

Index

Index